Table of Contents

Acknowledgements

When you share your voice and pen it down, you need a partner-in-crime who understands you, who reads your drafts, gives you advice, looks after your children, plays with them, feeds them, (and you and your pet) or orders take out. I could not have asked for a much better partner than my husband, Pratik. Thank you so much, dear. You are the best!

Writing this book has been quite a journey! It all started with Jami asking me to present a talk at her retreat and my talk and the impact it created on people at the retreat stuck with me enough to write a book about it. So I want to thank Jami, the spiritual goddess and my soul sister who brought this message from within me out in the world. Thank you for inviting me to rise up and share my voice.

To Aditi, my editor and my book coach, without you this book would never have been published! I am grateful for your gentle nudges, your keen insight and ongoing support in making my dream come true. It is because of your efforts and encouragement, I can call myself an author today! I am forever indebted to you.

To my parents Prabhakar and Rajani and my sister Shraddha and brother in law Ashish, thank you for always showing me how to live with light and prosperity in dark times.

To my children Riishab and Nihaal. It is because of you, I strive to be a better person every single day of my life. I hope that this book creates a legacy to pass on to our family and helps you find your prosperity as you grow up to be mindful adults.

To my aunt Leela, thank you for the encouragement you gave me in my early blogging days. You are no longer with us but your encouragement and blessings especially when I write are always felt. To my paternal grandfather Aba, thank you for showing me the importance of journaling every single day.

To my friend Sonal, you taught me forgiveness. For that I am forever grateful. You also posed great questions to me while pre-reading this book that gave me more insights on my own privilege and I am happy you helped me see that and keep it in check.

To Maru and Sean and to the entire team of speakers at Infinite Receiving Live, thank you for this event and for truly being a catalyst in my new life. I cannot go ahead with this book without thanking all my friends, mentors, coaches, teachers, and gurus who have appeared in my life, right when I needed them and have taught me appreciation towards humanity and our way of being. I am grateful to all my ambassadors, friends and people who have supported the launch of this book.

Without my wings, I will not be able to fly. You all are my wings that have supported me to fly when I took this giant leap of faith in writing this book. Thank you so much!

Praise For The Author

I have known Sneha personally for about 10 years now. When we first met little did I know that soon she would turn from an acquaintance, to a friend to a close friend and now my teacher and my guide. I have seen her evolve and grow in so many different areas of life, she has always been an entrepreneur at heart. I have seen her leave the corporate life and venture into her business for so many different ideas. I have always admired her strength and courage to try out new things and have always learned from her so much. It is from her that I learned to face my fears of money and uncertain future, it is from her that I have learned to dive into sound meditation, it is from her that I have learned to experience new things in life. I am forever grateful for our beautiful friendship and so happy for her. Congratulations on your first book Sneha, I am sure it will benefit a lot of people! I am looking forward to many more to come.

Namrata

Time with Sneha is a gift; and this book will allow so many people to receive that gift. I am fortunate to have spent the last couple years absorbing and enjoying the benefits of spending time with her, and it's difficult to put words to all I've gained. By learning to let go and practicing mindfulness, my life is much more full - full of gratitude, peace, acceptance and much more. I look forward to continuing to spend time with Sneha, progressing in my journey and I encourage you to pick up this book and do the same.

JC

I attended a couple of sound bath sessions with Sneha . And, the whole process seemed simple but quite powerful . Simple , since you lay down with your eyes closed and allow the various , unexpected sounds to help you relax. Powerful because it helps reach a state of awareness. I also did take a few coaching sessions with her when I was going through a rough phase in my life. I am thankful to have made that decision every single day . I have come out to be a different person in a better way - happy and positive towards life . Thank you Sneha for the work that you are doing and making lives better!!!

Manjari

I have been working with the beautiful and spiritually gifted Ms. Sneha for over a year and half. From day 1 until now her loving and caring healing energy has assisted myself and (5) five of my closest friends in clearing negative energy from our past, seeing what's possible for our future and finding our purpose in this lifetime. I am a loyal fan and consumer of Ms. Sneha work. I highly recommend any service Ms. Sneha has to offer. Ms. Sneha is AWESOME!!!

Tamara (Tammi) Edwards

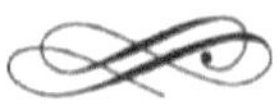

Feel supported in your
Stress Free Prosperity Journey

If you would like support, additional resources, and to connect to a community of people learning to ease their stress on the way to abundance and joy, please join us at https://stressfreeprosperitybook.com

Chapter 1

Never in my wildest dreams did I imagine that I would write a book on stress and prosperity. However, looking at my journey in life to date, I feel that I was meant to be the guide to help you understand how stress and prosperity are linked, making stress free prosperity the perfect subject to handle in my first book.

The impact of stress plays a major role in people's lives. The estimated cost to the global economy due to depression and anxiety is US $1 trillion per year in loss of productivity, according to the World Health Organization. Eastern Kentucky University estimated that American employers spend $300 billion every year on health care and lost work days linked to work-related stress.

Stress has played a major role in my life too. I have been through my fair share of stress due to accidents, surgery, heart breaks, career setbacks, entrepreneurial setbacks and more. And on that journey of navigating stress, every time I found a way to bring myself back on the road to prosperity.

The idea of this book is not to send you down the road of positive thinking your way to prosperity or denying your feelings and forcing yourself to feel positive. The idea of this book is to give actionable strategies to help you manage the pressure you feel and empower yourself on your path to creating wealth and lasting joy.

Who am I and why am I writing about stress and prosperity?

Hi, I am Sneha. I am a certified life coach, a certified mindfulness teacher and in the process of achieving my 200 hour yoga teacher certification. I wear many hats under the umbrella of StressLessWithSnehaJ.Com, a website I created to help busy professionals find the balance between joy and prosperity.

Throughout my life, I have been fascinated in understanding why adults are so stressed, about prosperity and personal growth, and the different ways to help them. To that end, I have found many mentors who have shown me the path to discover the way to being comfortable in my personal growth, every time I feel lost.

What does Prosperity Really Mean?

The dictionary definition of "to prosper" is to be financially successful. The word is also used to describe "to grow strong and healthy, to flourish physically."

Prosperity is your ability to *feel* that you are thriving, to know that you are doing well and everything that is happening is in your best interest and that you are growing. ***Therefore, prosperity is a state of mind, rather than your bank balance, or job title.***

Stress and Prosperity : What Is The Connection?

Stress and Prosperity are two sides of the same coin. When you see one face up, you do not see the other.

When you reduce stress in your life, you start increasing prosperity. Your outlook towards life changes. When the stress in your life increases, your feeling of control goes down.

Most of us play this coin flip all our lives. Something good happens and you get excited. Then something bad happens, and you feel that the world is just not supportive enough, and that you are not good enough. You start blaming everyone else including your stars and alignment, your parents, and partners and sometimes even your children.

You blame your work, your colleagues, your timetable, your health routine, and your bosses. Also, many times you blame yourself and you make a subconscious choice to continue to dwell on this blame game and you sit there whining. This causes you to feel less prosperous, since you are focusing on what you do not have.

But on the flip side, when you feel well in your mind and soul, you feel joyful. You do not feel the burden of stress on your shoulders anymore. You feel as light as air.

The difference between people who experience less stress and more prosperity in their life from those who don't is that these people are the ones who do something about it and learn when to adapt to situations or how to return to the balance.

I am not saying there are days where you will not groan from the pressures. I am not saying being upset is bad. I am saying knowing when to quit whining and take action changes your game in life.

And this is the hack that I want to teach you.

I will teach you how to *feel* more prosperous, more joyous and more happy in your life, while making sure that you unburden all that is not needed.

Is this magic? No.

Am I going to teach you some random "woo woo" principles about the law of attraction where you keep praying that you get more money to be prosperous? NO! I am going to give you a practical step by step process of how you can achieve more prosperity in your life and how to reduce stress in your life.

When most people think of prosperity, they start and stop at money, assets and wealth. But do you think that if you had tons of money and a lot of stress, you would be able to savor your progress 100%?

It is not possible, because with financial prosperity comes added responsibility and THAT reduces our ability to be calm.

Now, money is one of the factors that can help achieve prosperity but it is not the only factor. We have several factors in our life that affect how stressful or how prosperous we feel. In this book, I refer to these factors as the "Houses of Prosperity."

Houses Of Prosperity

To understand these houses, you need to be on the outside looking in at the various factors that affect your well-being. Each of these factors can be grouped into the following Houses of Prosperity:

1. Self/You
2. Relationships
3. Money
4. Space and Environment
5. Career/Purpose
6. Spirit
7. Network
8. Body
9. Time

The way you relate to each of these houses of prosperity can determine your prosperity at any given point of time. These houses can either make you feel good about yourself and your life or they may make your stress level rise.

Once we explore you learn about these factors; in the following section, I will take you down a simple path that will teach you a time tested, strategic process to achieve prosperity and lower stress in each of these houses.

My methods are a mix of practicality, science and wow! You have to understand how stress works, and how it affects your life. You have to get more clarity on what factors create a barrier to your prosperity. Once you have this clarity, you will be well on your way to stress-free prosperity!

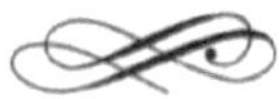

SECTION 1

HOUSES OF PROSPERITY

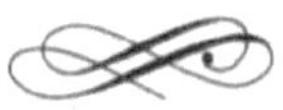

"Later that day, I got to thinking about relationships. There are those that open you up to something exotic, those that are old and familiar, those that bring up lots of questions, those that bring you somewhere unexpected, those that bring you far from where you started and those that bring you back.

But, the most exciting, challenging and significant relationship of all is the one you have with yourself. And if you find someone to love the you, you love…

Well? That's just fabulous."

Carrie Bradshaw (Sex and The City)

Chapter 2

When it comes to any relationship, I have always believed that the most important one is the one with yourself. The only way we can have a better relationship with others is if we have a good one with our own self. And that is exactly why the relationship with yourself is the First House Of Prosperity.

This house is ruled by self-care, boundaries, self-talk, and the mindset we build from our past experiences. For example, when I was considering writing this book, I needed to set apart time for myself to be able to do so. Writing a book is not a project that gives immediate returns, but I wanted to do it because I am passionate about the subject.

I knew that working on this project meant I had to take time away from some other daily activities and that there were some sacrifices that I needed to make.

In order to write this book and find time for it, I had to make sure that my priorities were communicated with those concerned. In my case, it would appear that I needed to communicate this shift in priorities with my family to ensure they understood that I needed to focus on my book and would not be able to perform some of the tasks in the household that they were accustomed to me performing.

Removing Self Doubt

Now if you were in this situation, you would have to ask yourself some questions:

- Would you be able to tell your family you needed time away from some of the daily family activities to write your book?
- Wonder if you are good enough to even write the book?
- Question if your message is important enough to be shared?
- Was this work important enough to prioritize over everything else?

I asked myself all of these questions. At times, I had to work on my mindset because I had to justify my self-worth to myself. I had to muster up courage and raise my self-esteem. I had to create boundaries between writing a book and everything else. In order to do this, I had to realize for myself that I needed to be true to myself first before I could be straight with my family.

How you show up for yourself in each of these questions will make you feel stressed or help you in achieving your goals.

Communication with Family

If you are easily able to tell your family about your needs with time, make a clear calendar, set boundaries, and move ahead with your project, you will feel free to express yourself the way you need to. If you feel that your message is strong, you will feel joyful and you will work on creating your work of art.

On the other hand, if you do not bring up your needs with those concerned, or if you decide to give in to your negative self-talk, then you will lock up your creativity which in turn will lock up the door to feeling abundant.

The most common stress trigger that most people have when it comes to their relationship with themselves is the feeling of not being good enough. This self-doubt shows up in various places throughout everyone's life. Most commonly it can show up as :

- self criticism
- low self worth
- self esteem issues
- feelings of rejection
- need for approval.

Your negative relationship with yourself will create a pattern of personal stress. Imagine that I did not have had the courage to raise my self-worth or overcome self-doubt? I definitely would not have felt confident to tell my family about my decision to write a book and set boundaries.

In order to establish a better relationship with yourself and feel prosperous, you have to work on changing your fixed mindset to a growth mindset. Establishing a growth mindset will help you move away from such issues, especially the need for approval from others.

Growth Mindset

According to Dr. Carol Dweck, a psychologist at Stanford University and the author of "Mindset: The New Psychology of Success," someone with a fixed mindset believes that their talents, intelligence and abilities are fixed and that effort is therefore a sign of inadequacy, while someone with a growth mindset believes that their talents, intelligence and abilities can be developed with effort.

When you have a more positive outlook about yourself, you naturally will open up your energies to create what you want in your life and in return open the door towards a prosperous life.

In this book, I want to give you basic strategies that can get you started on the way to a better relationship with yourself and thus help you get a better quotient in the first house of prosperity.

Growth Mindset Strategies

1.Challenge Negative Beliefs- Our beliefs are based on past experiences or values that have been handed down to us through generations. A lot of our credence is created in order to protect our ancestors, our families and us from perceived danger. But as time passes, these past beliefs become obsolete since we are no more in that situation. Naturally., we have to re-think these over time, mindfully.

- Ask yourself what you think about yourself
- Ask if what you believe is really true
- Ask yourself where you think this belief originated from
- Investigate your motive for this belief
- Rewrite a new positive belief about yourself
- Keep this new belief in your pocket or always visible to you

1.Look For Positive Evidence- Our brain is wired to look for evidence to support our beliefs. When you switch your negative belief to a positive one, it will take some time for your mind to adjust. Your mind will react like you are telling it a lie, because it may not be able to find evidence to support your new belief. This can propagate more self-doubt. When you look for and receive positive evidence for your new beliefs, your mind will start believing in them much freely.

2.Give Yourself Compassion- We are our own biggest critics. In our need for perfection, we create a greater struggle within. Giving ourselves the compassion we need to get through our daily lives is the key to opening up to prosperity.

Giving yourself compassion means to treat yourself like a friend, to say things to yourself like a friend would say to you in your difficult times.

3.Embrace Imperfections - We are naturally wired to constantly look at our imperfections first. Personally, this one was the hardest for me to change, but when it changed, it was truly life changing! The way to embrace imperfections is to stop focusing on external validation, societal standards and to move inwards, finding that inner compassionate voice. When we focus on giving value to ourselves first and then to others, all the talk (within ourselves) about imperfection dies.

With these growth mindset strategies, you are very well on your way to opening the doors of the First House Of Prosperity: Your Relationship With Self.

3 Simple Tips To Further Practice Growth Mindset

- Place positive beliefs as anchors throughout your workspace and house. You can use them as anchors when you feel down or distracted. Anchors are objects that serve as reminders of a central idea for you that help you enforce the particular idea. Pictures, vision board, sayings, wall art, T-shirts, computer wallpapers, bracelets, affirmation card decks all are examples of what can be used as anchors in your house. For example, I have placed a cork board with affirmations on specific positive beliefs I am working on embracing on the wall next to my computer desk. Whenever I am at my desk, I am reminded of my new beliefs.
- Make friends with people who are on a journey from a fixed mindset to growth mindset. It always helps to have company of similar thinking friends as accountability partners.
- Read books that help you enforce a growth mindset. I grew up reading books by Deepak Chopra, Tony Robbins, Eckhart Tolle, Sean Covey and more

Journaling Exercise

It is now time to put into action some of the strategies you have read in this chapter. I believe that when we put knowledge into writing and then into action then whatever we learned assimilates very quickly. You are welcome to use the space between each question to jot down your thoughts and answers.

1.What is a negative belief you are currently holding about yourself?

2.Where did this belief originate from?

3.How can you turn this belief into a positive one?

____

4.Write down 3 evidences starting today till whenever you find 3 to support your new belief about yourself.

____

5.Have you been hard on yourself about something today?

____

6.What would your friend say to you when you told them this?

7.Write down what they would say to you and say those words to yourself.

8.What anchors can you place in your house to remind you of your affirmations? Pictures, vision board, sayings, wall art, T-shirts, computer wallpapers, bracelets, affirmation card decks all are examples of what can be used as anchors in your house.

9.In what area do you feel you are not perfect? How can you embrace your imperfection today?

10.Which friend comes to your mind that may benefit or are already on a path of growth mindset? Can you connect with them and talk more about your process of growth?

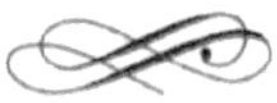

"It's not about how big the house is, it's about how happy the family is" Unknown

Chapter 3

Second House of Prosperity: Your Relationship With Your Family

L et's face it, the happier you are the more prosperous you feel. Many times how you feel about your family determines your happiness and prosperity.

The people who you care about the most are often the people who make you feel the worst about yourself. At the same time they are few of the closest people who can bring out the best in you as well.

Your daily interactions with your family are hands down the most important thing that determines how your day goes. Your family are the people who you start and end your day with. When it comes to familial interactions, we often fluctuate from loving to messy.

As a mother, wife, sister and daughter, I see the pendulum swinging on a daily basis. Kids go from being patient to not. Sometimes, as parents we go from being patient to not. And then there are times when we go from nurturing to wanting to be nurtured. When dealing with our spouses, we have to walk on eggshells at times, and others we can be completely open.

Clash Of Egos

When it comes to people, there can be competing needs. And this is equally true when it comes to people in the family.

Interestingly, as I wrote the first line of the first chapter of this book in my notebook and excitedly walked towards my husband to read it to him, I found him busy watching cricket. As I nudged him, he replied, "in 2 mins."

This made me really upset. After all, it was the first line of my first book. It was one of the most important things for me. I was shocked that it was not as important to him as it was to me. I wanted him to pay attention without any delay.

My brain started processing this very angrily. Thoughts such as, "Who does he think he is? How come my book is not as important as the thousands of cricket matches that people regularly watch!" raced through my mind.

I made some angry comments and walked out of the door. This in turn upset him. He banged the table. His brain processed everything very angrily as well. He spoke a lot of angry words, threw his wallet on the floor a couple of times, leaving me and the kids completely shaken.

The whole atmosphere in the room just changed in a flash. I went from elated to angry to scared. I started crying because I did not understand why he was mad when I was mad. I did not understand that it was not about cricket. My brain could not process the need for a person to have 2 minutes for themselves to finish the task at hand to be able to give another task their complete attention.

While this was something that was just a combination of misunderstandings that turned into a turbulence of emotions, this is not a very uncommon scenario amongst most people. We hear the words of our family, without understanding the process behind them, and interpret them in a much different way than intended.

When this happens, you balance the turbulence of emotions in a family with gallons of concoction of nurturing, understanding and compassion. It is how you will determine your emotional prosperity.

I suggest working on four focus areas that will help you create abundance of love, support and peace in this second house of prosperity:

1. Acceptance of familial shortcomings,
2. Working with your triggers,
3. Working on your emotional wounds, and
4. Creating boundaries

Let's look at these in detail here.:

Focus Area 1: Acceptance Of Familial Shortcomings

Often, family members are very quick to point out shortcomings of others. This is not done by your family to make you feel bad, but in order for you to correct your ways. Or you may have the habit of correcting others all the time or struggling to understand the shortcomings of members in your family.

In this scenario, I want to suggest using acceptance as a way to integrate the messiness of others and open up to new possibilities of being at peace. As parents, it is stressful to accept the shortcomings of our children.

For example, I have seen how hard it is for my child to accept change. This drove me crazy for the longest time. When I realized that this was something that made me feel impatient, I asked myself "what if I could stop fighting the way my child behaves?" Instead of trying to always change him and forcing him to feel ok, could I consider that it is his nature to be a little uncomfortable in making changes? Could I give him that extra time to adjust to new environments?

This question of acceptance helped me feel free from the constant worry I had. This freed up a lot of brain space for me and helped me become a more patient parent.

How can you implement this acceptance in your family?

1. Find one thing that you are constantly worried about or irritated about that one of your family members does.
2. Ask yourself this question: Can I accept this as a part of this person's personality, giving them space to handle this situation in their own time?
3. If the answer is yes, you will be able to give them space. If the answer is no, we come to the next focus area of how to deal with our family members.

When you bring this sense of compassion in your life and especially in your family, you will find more peace and acceptance in return.

In life we are all looking for reassurance and acceptance. When that reassurance and acceptance comes from our family, first, it means a lot more.

Focus Area 2: Working With Your Triggers

There are times you are triggered by your family and acceptance is not something that comes easily. You are triggered enough to be angry, upset, feel jealous, or worried. Leaving triggers unaddressed may lead to more hurt in your relationships. Let's understand what triggers are and how to heal them.

What are triggers?

Triggers are events or experiences that can prompt an inappropriate or overstated emotional reaction in a person as a result of re-living a traumatic experience by that person, mostly unknown to the doer of the action. Triggers lead to reactions that are upsetting and can lead to relationships being destroyed in extreme situations.

When it comes to triggers, I love to work with them in two ways:

1. I try to change the reaction I may have to the trigger so that I can stop further escalation which might make matters worse.
2. I try to understand the root cause of the trigger.

Changing the reaction to the emotional trigger

Our emotional triggers can be many. In neuro-transformational coaching with my mentor teacher and coach, Sean Smith, I learned that our emotional triggers are caused due to our judgement towards an event that occurred. We react based on our judgement towards the event , and not just the event.

Event → Judgement → Reaction

We need to learn to change our judgement to the event in order to change our reaction.

Event → New Judgement → New Reaction

So if you are not comfortable about your reactions to certain triggers, I now invite you to change the judgement towards these triggers.

I began using this strategy when my children were younger and I was a more vulnerable mother. One morning, I woke up super excited to go see my kindergartener get on stage for a certification with his school principal and have breakfast with him. This was a school event to recognize kids who show kindness and leadership. I wanted to witness a proud moment in his early life (his first month of kindergarten) and shower him with love.

Instead, my younger son who was then 3 years old, woke up cranky. He did not want to go with us to his older brother's school at 8 am and didn't want to go back to bed either. When I asked him if he wanted hot chocolate, he said yes. So I thought "Ok, problem solved!"

As he sat to drink the hot chocolate, his hand knocked the cup and a second later, the entire hot chocolate was on the floor. At that moment, we had only 15 mins left before we had to leave to go to my older son's school. and I still needed to get ready . So, instead of going to school with my kindergartner, I had to say goodbye to him and my husband. I stayed back and cleaned up the mess along with dealing with a cranky 3 year old. I had to miss the school event that I was so proudly looking forward to for days.

It was an excellent opportunity for me to have an outburst. I wanted to yell at the top of my lungs. I wanted to scold my 3 year old son for spilling the entire cup of milk on the floor. I wanted someone to soothe *me* because I was upset for not being there for my older son.

All I could think was "What if he thinks I do not love him enough? What if he thinks I favor the younger child more? What if he hates me for life for missing that event?"

But instead, I decided to change my *what ifs* in the moment. I decided to instead tell myself that it is ok. There will be a lot of opportunities in the future where I can be there for my son in person. It is normal for kids to feel disappointed but I can make him understand when he is older.

This new judgement put me into a state of calm. I took my 3 year old in my arms, gave him the compassion he needed and then put him to bed again so he could wake up fresh.

Understanding the root cause of the emotional trigger

Sometimes changing the reaction to the trigger can help us deal with a situation better and find peace . But other times, we have to dig deep beyond our judgements to find the root cause.

If you are triggered by someone in your house, you can ask yourself these questions and try to find the root cause of the situation.

1. If I am feeling upset because of this situation, what judgements am I placing on myself?
2. What beliefs am I carrying from my past that are being questioned in this moment?
3. Am I called to change these beliefs?
4. In which ways, am I forgetting to nurture myself in this moment daily?
5. Is there a past wound that is being pointed at because of this current trigger?
6. What can I do to heal this emotional wound?

Focus Area 3: Working With Your Emotional Wounds

Emotional wounds are past experiences that our subconscious mind carries in the present and believes them to be true. They are the result of an emotional trauma and skew our perceptions of the world around us. These wounds can create trouble in having a positive relationship with ourselves and others. We can categorize these wounds into four different types:

1. Rejection
2. Failure
3. Abandonment
4. Betrayal

Wound of Rejection

Growing up you might have faced some form of rejection. Maybe you were not selected in a sports team. Maybe you faced rejection from a group of friends and felt left out. Maybe you expressed your love to someone, and they rejected you.

How These Wounds Shows Up

- These wounds of rejection can show up in your life as a lack of confidence, or as a desire to stay invisible, or to voice your opinion less.
- You may keep yourself away from opportunities for the fear of getting rejected again and again.
- You may stop making friends if friends rejected you or you may keep rejecting love from others for the fear of getting rejected in the future.
- You may stop stating your needs when you are in a relationship for the fear of getting rejected.

In order to establish a positive relationship with your loved ones, it is important to work with these wounds of rejection.

Here are 4 ways to look at rejection in a new light:

1. Look at rejection as a divine re-direction that is taking you to a

more aligned path.

2. A rejection does not mean a no to you as a person. It is not about you but it is about the person or opportunity itself that may not be currently aligned to you or your path. If you are taking rejection personally, understand that it is not a personal issue.

3. A rejection may also mean it is meant to happen when time is right and aligned.

4. A rejection may also be a protection message that wants you to be safe at this moment.

Look at ways you have felt rejected and see what lessons you learned. Understanding which of these four situations apply can help you soften the blow of rejection.

Wound of Failure

You are bound to experience some form of failure. When you do, you may feel less motivated to move forward in your path. You may feel humiliated and inferior.

How This Wound Shows Up

- A wound of failure can show up in your life as guilt or shame.
- It can create low self esteem issues, you find yourself criticizing yourself and keeping yourself small.
- You may not take up new projects on your own or hide.
- You may start thinking poorly about yourself.
- You may feel you are not enough.
- You may feel jealous or envious of others.

Failure just means you have been given an opportunity to grow. Failure simply means there is more work remaining to do in the path that you are on. It means you have to work towards better alignment.

Here are 4 ways to look at a failure in a new light:

1. Failure does not mean failure unless you have stopped trying.
2. Failure just means you have been given an opportunity to learn and improve in the future.
3. It means you need to do some more work to do in your path

towards better alignment.

4. Sometimes, no matter how much you try, you may not find success on one path. In those cases, understand that you have to take a different direction.

Wound of Abandonment

At times in your life, you may feel abandoned. You may feel like you were left all by yourself in situations where you needed help and support the most.

Maybe, you were young and your parents had problems that were so large that they could not take care of you in the way you wanted them to. Maybe, your siblings did not like you the same way your friend's siblings liked your friend, played with them and took care of them. Maybe, you felt abandoned by your friend in school, when your friend made friends with another kid.

How This Wound Shows Up

- You abandon your own self when you need yourself the most.
- You are not able to take a stand or make friends.
- You choose to be lonely even if you have an option to be with people.
- You feel anger and irritation towards others.
- You have feelings of lack, i.e., of not having enough.

Here are 2 ways to look at abandonment in a new light:

1. Know that if you feel abandoned by other people, they may have reasons to do so and they were choosing the best thing for them and even maybe for you.

2. Look at the best things that happened to you after that abandonment and in spite of this abandonment. Do you think that your life would have been better, the same, or worse if they had not abandoned you?

Count the number of people who have been there for you. It is easy to focus on abandonment, or what you don't have, but if you focus on the support you have received, you will know that there are always more people who have supported you.

If you keep feeling sorry for yourself, you will go nowhere but down in dungeons of scarcity and lack. If you instead find learning opportunities in your experiences, if you find gratitude in your experiences, you will find ways to bring yourself above the wounds.

Wound of Betrayal

If growing up, someone broke your trust, it is hard to trust anyone again.

How This Wound Shows Up

- This shows up as indecisiveness and lack of trust in yourself.
- It can also show up as being stubborn and stuck up in your path.

How to help yourself through this wound?

- In this case, acknowledge the pain that this broken trust has caused you.
- Allow yourself to feel the emotions of pain, suffering, anxiety, anger, frustration, shame, guilt and others.
- See if you can allow yourself to forgive the betraying party. Forgiveness does not mean, what others did is right. It means that you will not allow yourself to keep hurting yourself because of this issue ever again. It means you release the emotions attached to this situation so that you can move forward freely and without a burden.

Focus Area 4: Creating Boundaries

No matter how much we love our family members, we need boundaries in order to maintain our sacred space. Setting boundaries does not mean you are a mean person. It also does not mean that you will be less liked by other people. Setting boundaries means that you respect your time and energy. It means you have more energy to be present, at your work and in your life without having to deal with negativities. It means that you are protected from other people and their situations. It also means that they are protected from you and your sensitivities.

Don't worry if you have a hard time setting boundaries, it does not come naturally. I can attest to that from my own experience. I went from being a complete people pleaser to a person with better boundaries at work and at home.

It is an acquired skill. It will not be overnight but I assure you, if you focus on improving this area of life, you will master it in no time.

How to go about setting boundaries in your relationships

1. **Learn to say NO**

   Creating strong boundaries is an important trait of a happy person. A happy person is committed to their happiness. This helps them not only keep themselves happy but also helps them be of service to other people and respond better. If a person cannot say no and does things even if they do not want to, it will be more likely that they will react to situations or act out and feel unhappy. Learning to say no is not selfish.

2. **Respect your time and energy**

   We start doing things for others out of obligation instead of choice. Know that you have the right to focus on your time and energy first before you decide to give others in the family your time and energy.

3. **Verbalize your priorities**

   This can give us great courage in sharing space with our family and still feeling like we have our own power.

4. **Respecting other people's boundaries**

   The more space you give others to be themselves, the more opportunities you will have to get the space you need for yourself. I have seen that people are often frustrated by others' behavior and keep worrying about changing others. True happiness and prosperity comes by taking responsibility to change our behavior, our reactions. and our beliefs.

While I listed all the stresses of the family and how to deal with them, I absolutely want to highlight the prosperity that family brings.

In my family, we have me, my husband, my two boys and now an addition of a new puppy, Luna. During recent times (as I am writing this book we are in the midst of the COVID-19 and are mostly staying home),we have been closer to each other than we have ever been.

Our kids are more open about their feelings, their joys, and their opinions. We have spent this year uplifting each other, adjusting to everyone being home every single day 24x7. We have learnt to adjust to schooling and working from home and being each other's friends. We have learned to navigate our worldly stresses through mindful communication and giving each other our presence. I do believe being present for each other as a family is particularly important.

A great way to make others feel present and communicate mindfully is through expressing love in the form of five love languages.

Five Love Languages

In the book "The Five Love Languages," author Gary Chapman outlines the five ways, or languages, in which a person may express and experience love. Everyone has a primary and secondary love language. He uses examples from his counseling practice, as well as questions to help determine one's own love languages (yes, there can be more than one).

His theory is that people have specific ways in which they receive love and usually use the same ways to express their love. If you pay attention to how people love to communicate their love, you might be able to understand their expectations better.

In my experience, understanding love languages really helps change your relationships. It took me a long time to understand my husband and my children's love languages. But once I did, it completely turned around the way I communicated with them.

For my older son, his love language is gifts and words of affirmation. If I speak angrily with him, he gets more upset than my other child.

For my husband, his love language is acts of service and receiving gifts (but only electronics). He shares his love in those two forms and receives love in those two forms of communication. And mine are gifts and words of affirmation. So, for me, I started to worry when my husband did not communicate his love as much through words. I kept wondering why he is doing so much for me but not saying much with words at all.

The book helped me understand how he communicated love by doing thoughtful things like remembering things to buy what I forgot to put on the grocery list or doing the dishes or helping with the chores as a regular thing he does at home instead of a special Mother's Day thing.

Remember, our family does care about how we make them feel. And how effectively we communicate our love and presence to each other is what keeps the family feeling joyful, present, and prosperous.

Here is an exercise for you to put into action some of the strategies you read in this chapter.

1. What are some common triggers related to your family that stress you out?

2. Are you easily able to verbalize your priorities? If not, why is it so?

3. Do you allow others in the family to prioritize themselves?

4. When was the most recent time that you had a severe emotional reaction to something in your family? How did it go? What did you learn from it?

5. Do you have a problem saying no to other people? What happens when you say no? What do you think compels you to say yes every time?

6. Describe a time when you shared more compassion to a family member in spite of being triggered?

7. What are some ways you nurture each other in your family?

8. List a few scenarios where you disagree with a family member. Does this disagreement cause you pain?

9. Write down an event with your family member that triggered you? What judgement did you make about the event? Can you change this judgement and look at the event with a new set of lens? What does this new lens teach you?

---

10. What are some things in your life that you have considered as failures? What have you learned from them? How has what you learned improved your life further?

---

11. What are some positive beliefs you have about yourself?

---

12. Write down a list of your accomplishments so far. After writing, notice how you feel about them. What change do you see in your mindset?

---

13. Have you felt rejected ever in your life? Write down more about this incident. Note down your emotions, feelings and thoughts around this incident.?

---

14. Has anyone left you feeling abandoned? Write down more about this incident. Note down your emotions, feelings and thoughts around this incident.?

---

15. Write about a time in your life when you felt like you were winning in life? What were your emotions, thoughts, feelings around this time? What can you do more to feel this way regularly?

---

16. In what ways will you share your learnings from this chapter with your family to help them create boundaries in their life and take ?

---

17. Do you know the love language for yourself and your family members? If not, read the book and find out.

"Health is like money, we never have a true idea of its value until we lose it." Josh Billings

Chapter 4

Third House Of Prosperity: Your Relationship With Your Health

This quote from Josh Billings in the previous page nails it. I never understood the true value of health, until I had a health scare. In December 2012, I suddenly found myself in the ER for a gallbladder surgery. From the outside, I looked normal and healthy, but inside was another story. I was not doing anything in particular to take care of my physical, or mental health.

This visit to the hospital and the surgery that followed were one of the pivotal moments in my life. It made me realize the true importance of maintaining a better relationship with my personal health.

We are not living our lives fully until we take care of ourselves. I passionately believe that life sends us wake up calls in terms of illnesses.

Since the gallbladder incident, I have always worked on continuously improving my outlook towards health. At present, these are 4 focus areas that I recommend people to work on when they are working towards better health:

- Food
- Exercise
- Mindset
- Rest

You are what you eat. There are various books on what you should eat, how much, what you should not eat, what to avoid. There are numerous theories around eating.

I recommend you choose foods that you most intuitively are called to eat. Listen to your body and your personal needs. Everyone's body constitution is different. What may fit as a great idea to eat for me may not be a fit for you.

When it comes to food, my expertise lies in helping people understand their relationship with eating and their emotions. Emotional eating is experienced by 27% adults in their lifetime. On the other hand, 30% of adults decide to skip a meal.

Both emotional eating or and skipping meals may be a way of handling emotions as an adult. A lot of us went to school and learned good manners, some exercises, mathematics, arts, and sciences. But we never learned how to handle our emotions.

Instead of learning or knowing how to deal with our emotions or stress, we tend to turn to food.

My wake-up call

In my case, I realized this a little later in life. Skinny is healthy is a big misconception. I was naturally thin looking, and I never really knew that I was binge eating and it was affecting me.

Until I found myself in an emergency room with an unexpected gallbladder attack.

They told me a person who undergoes gallbladder surgery is never as skinny as I was.

They were shocked. I was apparently skinny FAT.

The trauma of the surgery led me to a new path of looking at food in a whole new way. It was not immediately that I curbed emotional eating.

It took me years since then to become aware through a series of processes about how I handle my emotions and use food to self-sabotage my body and my health.

My certification journey in Mindfulness and Neuro-Linguistics Programming, as well as my weight loss plus mindfulness plus intentional intuitive eating journey, helped me understand how to handle emotions effectively. I learned how to become more aware of the emotional triggers I had. I understood how to deal with my emotions more maturely.

What is Emotional Eating?

Emotional eating is eating in response to difficult feelings when not experiencing physical hunger. It shows up as a craving for high sugar, high carbs, high-calorie foods.

Furthermore, people who eat emotionally tend to eat food to fill an emotional void. They also are known to connect food with their feelings, positive or negative. If you eat as a response to stress, you might constantly choose junk food over healthy food.

How to stop emotional eating?

The first step to stop emotional eating is to become aware of your eating tendencies.

Do you constantly find yourself reaching for sugar cookies? Do you tend to eat fast food a lot?

Are you in a state of constant worry?

Awareness is the key to solve any issue, especially emotional ones. Getting to know the triggers that cause you to pick the high-calorie food is essential next step. Learning how to handle your emotions and process them is essential.

As I mentioned earlier, we are not taught this in any school, house or social set up.

We have learned this by observing. And if we have not seen parents or our caretakers cope with their emotions healthily, there is a good chance we do not know how to solve this problem either.

In my 1:1 and group coaching programs, I teach my clients healthy ways to cope with the difficult emotions that they can use by themselves and also teach their kids and family. I also help them find healthy substitutes to their cravings and detoxing body from all the unhealthy substances that they have consumed.

It is always a good idea to visit your health care provider as well, to make sure you are not diagnosed with depression, bulimia or any other distinctive mental health disorders. In those cases, you will need extra help.

My experience and learnings have been most successful with people who have issues that can be dealt with mindfully. I recommend reaching out to your doctor, nutritionist, or therapist alongside my advice for personal growth.

Tips for Success in Curbing Emotional Eating

Accountability is key when it comes to finding success in curbing emotional eating. A coach like me, an accountability partner such as a spouse or co-worker, or your friends or family keep you from stuffing your emotions with food.

Finding and building a support system ahead of time is crucial. Ensure that your support system is more aware than you are, and if not, willing to learn to be aware of how to help you when the need arises.

Further, finding your bigger why helps. Acknowledging the main reason behind why you want to stop your unhealthy eating patterns will help you find the inner accountability and motivation to create new habits that take time to develop and stick.

What is mindful eating?

Mindful eating in its simplest definition is eating with awareness. It is an experience where you choose to eat with a moment-to-moment awareness. A mindful eating experience allows you to use all your senses in choosing to eat food that is satisfying and nourishing.

Having awareness while eating mindfully helps you understand when you are physically hungry vs. emotionally hungry. It can help you become aware of your current emotional relationship with food.

Most people eat mindlessly, in a hurry or exhibit a great degree of unconsciousness or indifference towards food. Usually, people eat with the television on and their mind switching between what is on TV to what is on their phones. Mindful eating gives an opportunity to bring awareness and attention to our bodies.

Here are 11 mindful eating strategies that will help emotional eaters change their experience around eating:

1. **Pay close attention to your emotions around food** – When you are eating a bite of food, close your eyes and tune in to your emotions around this bite of food. Ask yourself these questions. Are you attracted to this food? Do you feel in a hurry to eat? Are you annoyed to slow down and think about all these questions? Is there a sense of hatred towards this food? What are you hoping to get out of this food?

2. **Do not multitask**– While eating only eat. Turn off the TV, cellphone, computer. Do not talk to anyone else. Do not read.

Just give your complete attention to the food in front of you.

3. **Eat with a sense of gratitude–** When you eat food, think about what all activities must have taken place behind the scenes to get food on your plate. Thank the farmers, the industries, the chef, the logistics and transportation services, your ability to pay for the food, and pay gratitude to every little task.

4. **Slow down–** For the time that you are eating your food, slow down mentally. Try to not think about what you must complete next or where you have to reach. Just completely focus on food.

5. **Use all your senses–** Summon all your senses during eating. Truly work on smelling the fragrance of your meal. Touch the food and notice the textures. Does the food make a crunchy noise while biting or is it a soft chew? How does it taste on the tip of your tongue? What color is your food today? Is it appealing? Bring complete awareness to your food.

6. **Take 3 mindful breaths between some bites–** Put your fork down in between and take 3 mindful breaths. Then start eating again. This will help you bring you back from any distraction from this mindful eating activity back to the present moment.

7. **Notice how you feel after eating the food** – Do you feel satisfied? Do you feel nauseous? Do you still feel some form of a void? Do you feel full? Do you feel lethargic? Do you feel energized?

8. **What is your Hunger level?** Ask yourself how hungry you are on a scale of 1-10 where 1 is starving and 10 is full after a few bites? Repeat till you feel comfortable. Stop eating when you feel full and pack the remaining food for the next meal.

9. **Ask yourself why you are eating -?** Are you feeling stressed out or nervous? Are you feeling happy and excited? Are you feeling physically hungry?

10. **Use your non-dominant hand–** Use your nondominant hand to eat your food today. Notice how it feels. Does it feel awkward? Do you feel more aware of your eating? What is the judgment going on in your mind right now?

11. **Be mindful of what you are putting on your plate**– When you are choosing your food, ask yourself? Is this good for my body? Why am I choosing this food to eat right now? Will it help me feel better? Will it nourish my body? Do I usually feel crappy after eating this?

Mindful eating and becoming more aware of our patterns helps us to make changes. It will not help if we ask ourselves questions and go in a cycle of judgments towards ourselves.

Show self-compassion in this process as much as possible. Congratulate yourself on taking this important step towards becoming more aware of your eating patterns and emotions.

Here are some ways to succeed in using mindful eating process regularly

1. Put in your calendar to have one mindful meal or bite every day or every other day or every week or whichever pattern works for you the best.
2. Find a partner who is willing to do this with you and share notes.
3. Work with a mindfulness coach who will hold you accountable.

Exercise

My next favorite thing to talk about when it comes to health is exercise. When I lived in India, I was not aware of the importance of exercise especially how it mattered as I grew older. But even then, naturally we walked a lot. We walked far away to catch buses and public transportation. I remember walking for joy. I remember walking to go meet my friends.

That natural walking kept my body moving and fit in a lot of ways even though the awareness was not there.

When I moved to the US, my natural walking was replaced by my car. Cars are a necessary mode of transport in the US, especially for those of us who live in suburban areas, as things are widely spread and there is less access to public transit. Having to work out as a separate activity is a habit that I had to learn.

Next thing that changed due to this move was the introduction to foods from all over the world. I was so fascinated by restaurant foods that my normal homemade food was replaced by greasy cheesy take outs and we all know how that took a toll on my health.

Along with gaining awareness for food, I slowly changed myself and brought awareness of exercise in my life.

When it comes to exercise, I have the following mantras that I suggest:

1. Workout with a coach when you start so you get full benefit of understanding what is best for you.
2. Try a lot of things until you find out what is best for you.
3. Movement is the goal and any sort of movement you get to do, take that as a win.
4. Choose goals different than just weight loss. The reason I mention this is because when you choose weight loss as your goal, you tend to go off track as soon as you attain the weight loss you needed. And then you go back to the weight you had again pushing you into a vicious cycle of diet and temporary weight loss.
5. Focus on attaining strength and find your joy in working out.

Mental Health

There is a lot of stigma still around mental health. I do believe that taking care of our emotional and mental health is more important than physical health and should come first. Exercise and food help a lot in supporting mental and emotional health.

Getting support from therapists, coaches, and energy healers can be a great idea. All these categories of people have different strengths that everyone can benefit from. Make taking care of your health in all these areas a priority.

Mindfulness is a recommended practice. It is a quality of being — the experience of being open and aware in the present moment, without reflexive judgment, automatic criticism or mind wandering.

Mindfulness starts with becoming aware of your present moment and ends with understanding empathy, compassion, and self-love. When I came across mindfulness, I loved the simplicity of the practice. It was the easiest form of practice that I could have ever imagined.

Studies have shown these techniques to be an important tool to be used in helping cases of depression and anxiety.

As a mindfulness teacher, I recommend starting a mindfulness practice of 5-15 minutes daily and then extending it to longer times. Working with a coach will help you answer all your questions around the practice and yield great benefits when it comes to your mental and emotional health.

Rest

In today's times, people are constantly on the move. Everything is 24x by 7. If we are not in front of our computers working, then we are attending to our children, or running errands, or doing chores. When was the last time you shut everything down, put your feet up and just did nothing?

When we are stressed, our sympathetic nervous system (fight or flight response) is fired. As a result, stress hormones are created in our body. While this response helps in times of danger, a highly stressed environment keeps the sympathetic nervous system continuously fired up without going into a relaxation response or the firing of a parasympathetic nervous system.

This results in increased stress hormones in our body. The firing of relaxation response can help decrease stress hormones in our body. Due to chronic stress, the relaxation response fails to work on its own. You can read more about this in Dr. Herbert Benson's book The Relaxation Response.

It becomes our responsibility then to induce relaxation responses in our body through external measures.

Restorative Yoga, Mindfulness, Breathwork, Yoga Nidra and Sound Healing are some of the external tools I use for me and my clients to help reduce stress and promote rest and relaxation.

In today's world, it is easy to find these classes in nearly any location near you. In fact, you can also take part in some of these programs through online instruction. On my website, you will find a number of ways you can learn these with me in person and help you to be stress free.

Some easy ways to promote rest in your day-to-day life is by

1. Having boundaries between work and your life
2. Getting 7-8 hours of sleep

3. Not drinking caffeine after 2 pm in the evening
4. Building a daily meditation practice
5. Connecting with nature
6. Asking for help where necessary
7. Delegating
8. Taking breaks between work

Incorporating self-care in your daily life is key to having a healthy mind, body, and spirit. It is also the key to your prosperity.

Journaling Exercise

Here is a journaling exercise for you to immediately put into action some of the strategies you read in this chapter.

1. Do you eat when you feel stressed? What are some foods that help you feel nurtured?

2. What is your daily exercise activity goal?

3. Write down 5 things you can do on a weekly basis to help you focus on self-care.

4. Are you able to relax naturally? If not, what are your go to methods to induce relaxation in your body and mind?

5. How are your sleep patterns? Do you sleep 7-8 hours? Is your sleep peaceful or disturbed?

6. What are some of the stress thoughts that bother you daily?

7. How many glasses of water did you drink today?

8. How much caffeine do you drink?

9. What are some of your favorite fresh foods?

10. What is the biggest hindrance in your daily meditation and mindfulness practice?

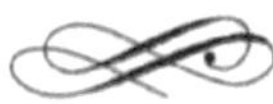

*"When I chased after money, I never had enough.
When I got my life on purpose and focused on giving of
myself and everything that arrived into my life, then I
was prosperous."*

Wayne Dyer

Chapter 5

Fourth House Of Prosperity : Your Relationship With Your Job and Purpose

Almost every person who has been put on this earth is either striving for a great job opportunity or looking for their purpose, or both. There are a few who do not care and live life unconsciously throughout their human life. Some are already living their passion or working on creating a great career.

The most common mistake I see people doing is thinking that their paying job must be their purpose or find purpose in their job. They then are upset about their job because it does not lead them to living with purpose.

To add to this feeling, people are stressed out at their jobs overworking, feeling undervalued and at the same time feeling the imbalance between work and home. This makes them feel unfulfilled, thus sad.

My friend called me one day and said she was stressed out at the job she used to love. She said, "I became a monster if I was getting late for my work." She felt bad for the loss of energy that happened because of tight schedules and the pressure.

She ended up quitting, then she went on a vacation to clear her head. She came back and now the reality of not having that job that she loved had hit her. She was not sure what to do.

She was able to go back if she wanted. She could find a new job. She could stay home. Unlike most people who do not have this open option, she had a lot of options she could choose from. This is what stress-free prosperity is all about.

Most people are always at choice point. They just forget that they have the options.

My friend loved working and her family equally. The pull of wanting to be there on both sides had become hard for her to bear. What she was looking for, was her dreams to come true and at the same time keep her family life in balance.

When she was feeling stressed, she had forgotten that she had a choice as well. A choice to make the ask, work the hours she wanted and not work during the hours she wanted to focus on her family.

When I gave her this suggestion to write down in her journal clearly what she wanted her job to look like, her eyes were opened to this new reality and she made the ask. She was offered a position in the workplace she loved exactly how she wanted her profile to look like. All her problems were solved. She felt good about both her family and her work.

What she did was instead of focusing on the money she made at her job, she decided to define for herself what prosperity meant for her. For my friend, prosperity meant being 100% present at the place where she was at. Being overworked and exhausted did not let her be 100% at home with her children. So, she redefined prosperity to mean taking a job that would let her be present, with her family, when she was home.

I could completely relate to her quest of prosperity and I am glad that this worked out for her. My quest did not exactly begin in the same way and my story is entirely different, but I have been in this tug of war before. I have found myself at a crossroads of job and higher purpose. I have wondered if my job should take me to my purpose, or if there should be more than what I have been working with, if there should be a balance in my life.

For me, the path was entirely different. My path required me to do more soul seeking to find out my purpose that gave me more joy. At that time, I decided to focus more on my children and let go of the financial responsibility completely. This helped me focus on learning what I always wanted to learn and explore, and at the same time lowering the family burden from my husband's shoulder. He had to take complete burden of the finances, but with me being happier, our life ended up feeling more prosperous than before when we both made more money.

Maybe you, who are reading this, are facing a tug of war as well. Many times, you face this tug of war when your value systems that you, yourself have not yet fully recognized, are challenged to the core.

While writing this, I do acknowledge my privilege and the privilege of my friend. We both had the choice of quitting our jobs and being financially dependent on our better halves until we figure out life.

Not everyone has that option and I very well recognize that. And with that recognition, I believe that no matter what cards life has presented you with, you always have the opportunity to work on your purpose by getting very clear on your personal values and aligning your actions with those values in the best way you possibly can.

The Road To Hell Is Paved With Good Intentions.

Severe stress happens when what you want and the value of what you are doing is at a crossroads. Regular incidents like these can lead to burn out.

Therefore, it is a good idea to examine intentions and values at regular intervals.

When you are working at a job, understand your intention behind the job. Are you working because of the passion you have for your job? Are you working because you have a financial responsibility? Are you working because just being out of the house gives you joy and meaning?

Knowing this and becoming mindful can help you not look for something in your job that it is not meant to give. If your job solely provides you a means to live and nothing else, then it is ok to do that as long as you recognize this and not try to derive purpose from it.

If your job is meant to serve a higher purpose and not just provide you with financial independence, then you can examine it further.

Does your job meet your values? If your primary value is your family, then is working overtime regularly at your job meeting that value for you? If your primary value is personal growth, is you working at your job giving you that.

You find stress-free prosperity at your job if you look at it in either one of these two ways:

1. Your job and your purpose are aligned. You feel valued where you are working, feel that this is what you were born to do, or
2. You know your job and purpose are different, you have enough time, energy and resources to devote to each of them to have perfect harmony.

The issue arises when you don't feel aligned to your job or you don't get enough energy and time to devote to what you think you were born on this earth to do, or when you try to derive purpose from your job but your job is not designed to give you that.

Finding this alignment is important.

Identifying Your Purpose

Our values guide us. When we know and honor these values, we truly experience fulfilment.

When we do not accept our values, we possibly meet stress on the way more often than not.

A lot of times external values are imposed upon us by our upbringing, media, politicians, our religion, and our workplaces. Most people live their life not knowing what really mattered to them the most.

Here are a few steps to identify your values in a mindful way:

A guided classroom experience is best suited for this example which is part of my mindfulness course but I will give you steps to try this exercise at home.

Step 1: Sit in a relaxed posture with your back straight. Meditate quietly focusing on the breath. Do not alter your breath. Do not focus on the thoughts. Just focus on the incoming breath entering the nostril and outgoing breath leaving the nostril. Allow yourself a few minutes in this state that will help you prepare for further contemplation.

Step 2: Now imagine you are nearing the end of your life and have just finished writing your autobiography and are considering a "moral of the story" or "a message for the end of the story." There is no need to get threatened or afraid. Consider your values and successes. Now forgive your humanity and consider how you could have better lived those values. What could you have done better for others from this future place?

Step 3: Imagine this future self-talking to the present you. What would he/she say? What is your meaning in life? What is your true purpose? How can you better fulfill your purpose?

Step 4: Come out of this meditation space and take a sheet of paper and write down your life's purpose. Write down what core values reflect this. For example, if your purpose is to improve the lives of others, you might write compassion, generosity, etc. If your purpose is to travel the world then you might write freedom, prosperity, connections, etc. Refrain from judging your purpose. Also write down intentions that come from the knowledge of your purpose and values.

Step 5: Affirm these core values in a mirror. Tell yourself what your purpose is, what your values are, and how you will be those values in action.

Step 6: Really look at your purpose and your intentions and bring into mind one intention. Examine it. See what may stand in the way. Become aware of your strengths and the needs for the intentions to be met.

Does the intention truly increase the greater good? Make sure your intention is sound. Now take the first step towards fulfilling the same.

Identifying our purpose and staying on the path to fulfill it minimizes our stress in a lot of ways. Your current job may or may not be something that is the same as your purpose. If it is not, you can either focus on finding a job that is more aligned with your purpose, or you can use your spare time, such as time you might have used to watch television, YouTube, or something else less valuable you devote your time to in your life, to fulfill your purpose.

I hope you get more clarity on your path as you embark on this journey of moving from careers that cause stress to living a more purpose filled life and career.

Cautionary Note

I wanted to share a cautionary note. A lot of people waste time running behind finding their "passion" or asking around for their purpose. Instead, follow fulfillment. Whatever makes you feel whole, full of energy, happy and joyful, do that. When you start sharing value to the world from this place, passion and purpose will meet you and find you right where you are.

Here is a journaling exercise for you to immediately put into action some of the strategies you read in this chapter.

1. Do you know your core values?

2. Do you know what your purpose is? Did you go through the purpose meditation exercise? Did it help you get more clarity on where you need to focus more?

3. Does your job give you joy and satisfaction?

4. Do you have hobbies or volunteer work or creative outlets that give you more satisfaction than at your workplace?

5. How much time in a week can you dedicate to doing what you value the most?

6. What changes do you need to make in your routine to give your purpose a priority?

---

7. Does your current lifestyle fit the path to your purpose? If not, what changes do you need to make for it to fit?

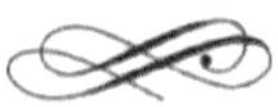

"Happiness is a place between too little and too much." Finnish proverb

Chapter 6

When it comes to space, there can be three kinds:

- Mental,
- Physical, and
  - Energy

Since we have discussed mindset, relationships, and physical health in previous chapters, in this particular chapter we will focus on our physical space.

Your physical space is the space where you work, sleep, eat, create, and take a breather. This could be a combination of your house, office, car, desk space, kitchen, etc.

A 2009 study shows that women with higher stress home scores (stress = with clutter or seemingly unfinished) were more likely to suffer from depression as compared to women with higher restorative home scores.

Pause reading for a moment, and give a good look around the room you are currently sitting and reading this book in. Do you enjoy this space? Do you see clutter? Do you immediately think of a list of to-dos as you look around? Or do you just see beauty and love? Does it give you more light and energy or does it suck all enthusiasm away from you?

Now close your eyes and see with your mind's eye. What do you really want this space to look like? What purpose do you want it to solve for you? Do you want this room to be light and airy, and full of inspiration? Or do you want it to be a place that lets you rest and sleep?

Here are some problems that I often see:

1. If your office is full of to-dos and reminders of different tasks, then your desk will not be the space where you can focus and do one thing. You will be constantly shifting your attention from one thing to another.

2. If your kitchen is full of empty containers and not well stocked, you will always be calling in food.
3. If your living room is full of clutter, it will not be a place for you to sit down and relax and read a book and never a place for you to welcome guests.
4. If your bedroom is full of clothes that need to be folded, it might not be a place for you to connect with your partner or have good night's rest.

What this can further lead to is

1. Frustration
2. Procrastination
3. Loss of Focus
4. Loneliness
5. Restlessness
6. Anger
7. Emotional Eating and more

Best Practices for Healing Your Space

Here are some best practices for some areas of the house that I have worked on that help me feel sane on most days.

Laundry

A lot of people get worked up about laundry. This is one area where I have mastered by adjusting my life accordingly. When the laundry washing and drying cycle is going in my house, this is what we are doing:

- Immediately folding clothes as soon as we take them out of the dryer. I have timed this, and it takes 15 mins per basket to fold (Did I tell you I was an Industrial Engineer in my previous life and process improvement involved timing a lot of processes?!)
- Fold as a family or at least both parents and not just the mother or father.
- Everyone keeps their own clothes back in their own closet as soon as they are folded. Kids as well.
- Whatever that needs to be ironed still goes on hangers and is ironed as needed or sent to the dry cleaning and ironing place. A lot of times we outsource adult ironing. This was a no brainer when we

grew up in India but if we are to save our time in the day this is where we save it.

Kitchen

In the kitchen we have tasks divided.

- I cook, and my husband cleans the dishes. I put the clean dishes away.

- I make the list, my husband buys groceries or picks them up and I put them away in their place.

- This makes me accountable to know what I bought, how much is left, and I ensure that things are in their place and in stock but it does not overwhelm me or take my energy away as I do not have to physically go and buy it myself.

- I trust my husband to take care of things he is responsible for. Reducing each other's burden takes a lot of overwhelm away.

- In the pantry, I have areas divided by type of food like grains, proteins, breakfast area, cans, pastas, snacks, etc. I have a separate area for spices, separate areas for tea coffee sugar.

- My utensils and gadgets are divided by utility.

- In the refrigerator, we try to use up things before we add new things to it.

- We do not buy what we know we will not use. And that sometimes limits the range of foods we eat but we know that we can count ourselves on reducing food waste in the house.

Living Room

Our living room is set in a way where we have seating arrangement in a U shape with a coffee table and these are all facing towards the TV and fireplace and wall cabinets. One of the major sources of stress is our kids bringing toys, books and paper, and adults bringing mail and all this keeps collecting on the center coffee table. If I have to generalize, I will say the most pressing issue in the house has been flat surfaces and keeping them empty and minimal looking instead of piles of messiness. This does not only cause stress, but it has also caused me frustration and anger and has made me lose my mind a multiple times. The way we have started handling this is by:

- Finding a place for everything and making sure we keep everything in its place.
- A definite place for incoming mail and in process mail.
- A specific place for toys and playing, drawings and coloring/art related activities.

As a parent, I get the messiness.

Mess is often out of control and too much to manage. Especially, if you are planning to tackle this all by yourself. That is exactly where most of the problem lies. Everyone in the family is involved in making clutter but it affects one person more than the rest. This person makes it his/her personal responsibility to clear it out and gets overwhelmed and drained. And other times the mess is caused by just one or two people in the house and these people are completely oblivious to this fact, but it bothers everyone else.

In either scenario, instead of making clearing clutter one person's responsibility, make it a task for the entire family to divide and conquer.

The most important part to remember though, is that to not let the mountain of responsibilities of clearing a space overwhelm you. Instead, focus on the area you are using for the day and give it your intention, energy, and love and it will give you the energy, transformation and healing that you need from the space.

Even though our space can give us stress, it can be the very container we need to express and feel joy.

I love putting up decorations according to the season. I love enhancing the decorations with indoor plants (though some plants are toxic to my puppy and I have to be careful what plants I choose). Walls are a great space to share quotes that motivate you, share your culture with others, and create opportunities to spark conversations.

Every room should have an intention and decorated according to its intention. For example, if a bedroom is for relaxation and connection with your partner, then children's toys and electronics may not be the best pieces to go in that bedroom.

Your work room should not have a place where you are constantly reminded of your daily stressors. When you tackle each room and space with intention, you find that there is less you need to fill in the space and more room for what you most desire.

Here are some final points to remember and implement to have a space that helps you feel less overwhelmed and more prosperous

1. Create good habits of creating a place for everything and keeping everything in its place.
2. Make sure everyone understands that keeping the house clean is a team effort and not just one person's responsibility.
3. Create routine cheat sheets and reminders for young kids as well as adults to keep up with accountability.
4. Remember to set an intention for each space and then decorate or set it up accordingly so that its use is intentional and easy to clean up for the young kids as well as adults.

Journaling Exercise

Here is a journaling exercise for you to immediately put into action some of the strategies you read in this chapter.

1. How do you feel about your current space?

2. Which area in your house has the most clutter?

3. What about your environment bothers you the most?

4. What steps can you take to make changes to your space?

5. Have you decorated each room in your home or office with complete intention?

6. What decluttering tasks can you divide amongst your family members?

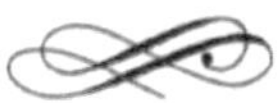

"Opportunity is missed by most people because it is dressed in overalls and looks like work."
Thomas Edison

Chapter 7

When it comes to your relationship with finances, the one thing I would love to say is you have to start with building a proper foundation. When people converse about money, they either talk about investments or assets.

I believe that even before we start talking about the technical stuff such as investments and cash flow, we must take care of our financial foundation. Finance is a very vast topic, and I am going to do my best to not get dragged down the rabbit hole by only touching on two major points in this chapter. Hopefully, these help you get started on a road to financial prosperity.

When it comes to a strong financial foundation, we must focus on two aspects.

1. Money Mindset, and
2. Practicality

I could write separate books on each of these topics (and others probably have), so I will try to keep the discussion high level in this chapter to help you get started in the right direction.

Money Mindset

When it comes to money, having a mindset that is conducive to strengthen your relationship with money is particularly important.

Our money mindset is molded to a large extent by our parents' money mindset, rather than by our own experiences with money. It is strange to think that instead of thinking about money based on things we have heard and learned, we do it based on what our parents learned and experienced. This may or may not be a good thing depending on your personal experiences and background. I feel that everyone can work towards improving their money mindset.

Here are 5 steps you need to take in order to work on

your money mindset:

1. Become aware of your money stories and your money beliefs. As a mindfulness expert, one thing I have realized is that awareness is key and the first step for anything you need to make a transformation in.
2. Now, out of these money stories and money beliefs, find out which ones are working against you and are not in favor of you having more wealth.
3. These are the beliefs and stories you will work on breaking the pattern and re-writing to a new story. You can do this through journaling, through EFT, through working with an energy healer or life coach who focuses on money.
4. The next step is to set new intentions and goals for your wealth. We have a chapter later on that focuses solely on intention setting.
5. Make all the above steps a regular habit to transform your money beliefs into more supportive ones.

Practicality

When it comes to finances it is important to take care of the basics. Every family needs 6 basics when it comes to finances.

- Proper Protection
- Debt Management
- Emergency Funds
- Cash Flow
- Building Wealth and
- Preserving Wealth.

What is a financial foundation?

Just like every house requires a foundation in order to stand stable on the ground, similarly, a financial house requires a strong foundation. A great financial foundation is where you have created a way to protect your family's assets and protect your family against loss of income.

Having a will and trust according to laws in your state and country helps protect your family's assets. You can get this done through an attorney or through some online services that provide documents that are accepted in some states where you can do the work yourself and save some attorney fees. It all depends on how complicated your life situation is. Make sure you talk to a legal and financial professional before you make this decision.

Having life insurance protects your family. A lot of families are not adequately protected when it comes to life insurance. There is a simple formula that you can use to calculate how much life insurance you need.

Life insurance is a transfer of risk. You must know how much your risk is. If you are a family person, your risk will be your debt, your annual income (times roughly ten so that your family can live comfortably for a few years until they figure out how to move forward without you in their life), your mortgage amount, and your kid's education needs. You must make sure that you take care of these risks and transfer the headache to a life insurance company.

I have seen way too many people that do not have insurance policies (or have insufficient coverage) who leave their family behind scrambling for paying mortgage and suddenly looking for jobs. You do not want to be one of them. Yes, your friends might create a crowd-funding page for your family, but it is only fair to not have your friends share the risk of taking care of your family even though they may willingly do it.

If you have a strong foundation, you will be able to eliminate at least one source of stress in your life. You will now have built guardrails on the journey of life, that will protect your family from falling off the bridge, and therefore give you the ability to drive with less care down the road of life.

Building further upon a strong foundation

- After building a strong foundation, one must take care of their debts and emergency funds. Debts build fast and we are on the wrong end of the rule of 72 when it comes to debts. The interest rates are high, and it takes no time for our debt to almost double up, if we do not take care of it sooner. The rule of 72 is defined as a rule of thumb to estimate the number of years required to double your money (or your debt) at a given annual rate of return (or interest rate in the case of debt).

- The next thing to work on is emergency funds. A minimum

of 3-6 months of your monthly salary should be saved up to help you in case of any emergencies.

- In today's age, it is also quite important to have a secondary source of income. You can start a business, get a second job, or monetize your passion. Whatever it is that you choose, with the given rate of inflation and uncertainty in the job market, having something on the side always helps. Yes, this can create a source of stress if you do not use your time wisely and balance all your houses of prosperity. So be sure this is something you really are passionate about and have the energy to take on before taking on extra responsibilities that will burn you out.

- Once you have taken care of all this, then you can talk about investment strategies, retirement etc. (the fun stuff).

- When it comes to retirement strategies, I believe in creating a monthly income goal avenue after retirement alongside building assets.

- A lot of people work only on assets but forget about creating an income for retirement. This leads to a lot of people outliving their savings wealth while they are still living and

- then are forced to work at hourly jobs later in their age and not live the best retired life they had hoped for.

The Importance Of The Value You Provide

A well thought out financial plan is the best plan. A lot of times, people fail to plan and then they fail in their financial house. My aim with this chapter was to help you open your eyes and start working towards a better financial future.

The last thing I want to talk about is using wealth as a tool. The idea is to focus on the value you provide through your work and services and focusing on how you can be valuable to the world.

Once you have this taken care of, money will follow you. This is the secret of financial prosperity. If you keep focusing just on money and not the value you provide, you may get a lot of money, but that money will only amplify the problems you have.

It is important to take care of financial issues at the foundation level for money to start flowing in. When you provide value, you feel more fulfilled and more prosperous than just processing empty wealth flowing in.

This trio of financial foundation, money mindset and the value that you provide to the world will take you to the road of financial prosperity and long-term wealth building and help you create a legacy for your future generations to come.

Here is a journaling exercise for you to immediately put into action some of the strategies you read in this chapter.

     1. Is your financial foundation strong?

     2. Do you have a particular financial goal for you and your family? Are you on track to achieving it?

3. What is your action plan to achieve this goal?

4. Whose help will you take to help your financial goal?

5. What are some of your positive money beliefs?

6. What are some of your negative money beliefs?

7. How will you rewrite your money beliefs to help you achieve financial prosperity?

8. Are you working towards creating a better future for you and your family by reducing your debts?

9. Are you saving for your retirement? Do you have a retirement saving goal?

10. Do you have a monthly budget?

11. Do you have emergency funds? If not, what is your plan to build those up?

12. Do you have a will and trust to leave your legacy to your family? If not, what is your plan for that?

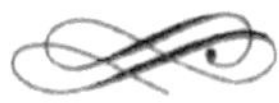

"Pulling a good network together takes effort, sincerity and time."

Alan Collins

Chapter 8

I am blessed with a really good network of people. When you are in the company of true people, you feel blessed, happy, and prosperous.

Friends, colleagues, neighbors, members of communities we are associated with, all add value to our life. And in a lot of ways, we add value to their lives. We get to learn about different perspectives, different cultures and different lifestyles.

When we get together with people, it also means there can sometimes be differences of opinion or arguments over something that you do not see eye to eye with. Differences of opinion are ok, as long as there is mutual respect. One needs to find the space to agree to disagree, or else your network can end up leaving you in stressful situations for days on end.

Believe it or not, in today's technology driven world, where networking is an important way to bond with people and grow in community, it can quickly become a headache to some. Competing with your network, feeling used by your network, feeling judged, and judging your network are so rampant in our communities that it becomes exhausting to be a part of larger communities.

Satsang is a Sanskrit word which means gathering of true people. Should our network gathering be a gathering of true people, of authentic people, or should it be a gathering of people keeping up with each other, gossiping behind each other's backs?

This is up to us to decide really on what we want from our network. Are you looking for a true connection, are you looking to spend your time in a productive manner and for the larger benefit of the society or are you looking for fuel for drama?

I see cultural gatherings and holiday celebrations as a way to get to meet new people, get to learn about new customs and just enjoy. I have also seen some cultural gatherings turn into sour relationships over misunderstandings, leading to exclusion of people from future gatherings.

Not just a gathering but in general, keeping up with the quality of life of our network can also become exhausting. A neighbor buys a new TV and suddenly you feel like buying one too. Someone invests in gold jewelry for their anniversary, and then you want to buy a gold necklace as well. Someone else has a pink dress that you like, and you want a blue dress in the same style. I see this kind of keeping up happening with children in school as well. If one friend has a skateboard, everyone else feels the pressure of owning a skateboard. If one friend has a pony, everyone else feels the pressure of owning a pony.

I believe in order for parents and children to stop falling into this pressure trap, there should be an emphasis on understanding personal and family values, interests and priorities. Focus should be on what lights the person, the child, and the family and not what others have that do not have. There is a lack mentality that is rampant in today's society. People are more envious of others instead of being happy for themselves and their own situations. This is what is commonly referred to as FOMO, or the "Fear Of Missing Out."

The envy is not a sign of true prosperity. Envy is a sign of a lack mentality. If she has it, I want it too. If he has it, then that means that I might not be able to have it. This leads to unfair competitions, backstabbing and more. All of which increase stress on one's life.

And all of us fall prey to this behavior. We have been always taught that there is room for only one at the top. But that is not true. We all have our gifts, and we can all find our way to *this metaphorical* top. We do not have to feel behind and lesser than, if we do not have something that others do.

I learned from one of my coaches, Maru Iabichela, that when you see someone else owning or getting something, you so desperately want, see it as a sign of evidence that you will have it soon as well. This will help you to send them a blessing for their achievement and be happy for them. This will help you to get away from the low energy of feeling envy and move you to a higher vibe. This lesson changed me a lot. I started appreciating women around me more. I always thought that there could be only one woman in a group, the "Alpha woman." There cannot be others. But this superior mentality is really just inferiority in disguise. Maru's lesson helped me understand, respect, to take help from and to help other women. It helped me save a lot of heartache and energy that I would have otherwise spent in jealousy and envy.

In my few years of meeting and growing my network, I have learned a few do's and don'ts that I will share with you below. I hope this will help you become valuable to and help you see value in your community as well.

Dos and Don'ts

1. Do not talk behind other people's back. This always backfires. Instead, be straightforward and share your problem along with a solution directly with the person involved. Before sharing a problem, always appreciate the other person and their efforts first. This will help them see your problem better and will not feel like they are being attacked. They may or may not take your suggestion but will appreciate you being direct.
2. If you are taking someone else's valuable time, be as precise in your ask as possible. Make sure you always give value first, before making an ask.
3. As much as I value inclusivity, exclusivity is part of networking. If others do not see you with the same values, you will be excluded. You cannot force others to include you and others cannot force you to include them. If you see exclusivity as an issue, remember you can always start your own circle and become more inclusive yourself. I teach this to my kids as well. There will always be times where others will not see you as their friend or you will not see others as your friend. That does not mean you become unkind or rude towards them. It just means that you will learn to be acquaintances. The clearer you are on who you are, the less exclusivity will bother you.
4. Measuring people with wealth is not always the right way to make friends. Yes, your network is your net worth, but your net worth is not everything. This again boils down to how clear you are on who you are and what values you live by.
5. Be kind, always. There is no point in being rude. Everyone has a right to their opinion and so do you. Share your point of view with respect and kindness. But do not let others take your kindness as your weakness. There is a thin line between kindness and being a people pleaser.

Here are 11 (yes, 11) ideas on where you can find like-minded people:

1. Meetup.com - When I lived in Las Vegas, I used this website primarily to meet new people. I was new in town and I knew nobody. I found real gems of people. You can find people based on matching interests. When we did not have children, we found a network of couples to hangout and party with. I met people from different strata of life, and my perspective on life changed a lot. Before that, I had not really interacted with people who did not have similar backgrounds or socio-economic status as mine. When I was pregnant, I found other pregnant women in other meetup groups and a lot of us became friends as our children grew up together (well until I had to move to Atlanta).

2. Yoga or Exercise community - I see a lot of people making friends through this way.

3. Workshops and classes, you take - Again people with similar interests can be found in places you go to learn together and you can become friends there and hang out more.

4. Community events

5. PTO events

6. Neighborhood events

7. Events at the places of worship

8. Volunteering opportunities

9. Workplace events

10. Entrepreneur Networking Events, and

11. Facebook groups - You can virtually hangout in different groups based on your interest and interact with people in the community.

Choosing the right network can bring you a lifetime of joy and prosperity. Remember, you always have a choice of who you want to meet with, be friends with and hangout with. The more you remember your values and that in all situations you have a choice, the happier and more prosperous you will be in all situations.

Here is a journaling exercise for you to immediately put into action some of the strategies you read in this chapter.

1. When you come home after meeting people, do you feel inspired or drained?

2. Do you feel good about yourself or do you feel superior or inferior?

3. Do you feel jealous and envious of the people around you or do you think they feel jealous and envious of you?

4. How does that affect your life negatively?

5. How clear are you on your and your family's values?

6. Write down the time when you had a great time with your network. What were you doing? What were you talking about?

---

7. Write down the time when you really felt out of place while networking. What were you doing? What was everyone talking about? How was your mindset then?

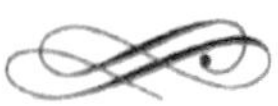

"Too busy is a myth. People make time for the things that are really important to them."

Mandy Hale.

Chapter 9

Eighth House Of Prosperity: Your Relationship With Time

Over time I have realized that the most finite thing we have in our life is time. We do not come on the earth with infinite time. When we are born, death is certain. We just do not know when.

We all run behind money and feel it is limited. So, we take a lot of time away from things we love and spend time on making money (or saving money). And making money and creating wealth is not a bad thing. But at the expense of what, is always the question.

The point I want to make is, we have limited time on earth. And when we have limited time on earth, it is our responsibility to make the best use of it.

I did not know this when I was young. I did not put too much thought into it. I let time pass by me. I did not take some things seriously like learning music when the time was right or letting go of hurt and forgiving people before it was too late. But as I am getting older and wiser, I have started taking my time more seriously. People say time is money, but time is so much more precious than that.

How you use your time will affect how stressed you are. Have you had a day where you were super busy, did all the things that you loved and felt wonderful at the end of the day? Now was there a time when you were bored, and did not do much other than watch TV all day and at the end of the day felt really stressed out?

I am not saying TV is bad and working too much is good. Yes, watching TV can be relaxing sometimes. And yes, too much work in a day can be stressful as well most of the time. What the above example means is, that when we feel aligned with the work we are doing, no matter how much time we spend doing it, we will feel less stressed. We can feel tired, but not mentally stressed. It will be easy to go into relaxation after working hard on our favorite projects.

When we are not aligned with the way we should be relaxing, we will feel the stress of it. Watching TV is relaxing for a few minutes and a quick fix, but it does not give the body the relaxation response that it really needs.

Our relationship with time is a skill that we need to master. And I am not just talking about productivity. There are many productivity gurus out there. I am talking about managing time so that your life feels balanced. And balance does not mean spending equal time on everything. It means spending time on things that matter the most.

Here are some ideas that I have implemented when it comes to time that are working for me:

1. The most important time management skill that I learnt the hard way is putting everything on a calendar time slot. This really helps to get things done. Sometimes, if you forget to regularly open the calendar and look, having a smart device can really help you keep up with your calendar and tasks.
2. I set an intention of completing one main thing, every day. When I prioritize one thing that needs to be done, it gets done. The maximum number of tasks that I prioritize is 3. If I commit to anything more than 3 tasks for a day, I know that I am going to fail and not get those things done.
3. I delegate things that I have no energy or time for. Sometimes, that could be cooking, cleaning, or something else. Especially when I am schooling kids at home due to COVID-19, have a new puppy, and business and clients to attend to. Outsourcing and delegating are the best ways you can make time for what you really care about. Asking for help is considered weak, especially here in the USA. I grew up in a family where we had a lot of help at home. Having help around the house is certainly not inexpensive here in the States, but there are times when help becomes necessary in order to focus on what is more important.
4. Becoming more mindful of where we spend time is the next most important thing. Time goes by fast when we scroll social media pages. Time goes fast worrying about things that have not happened yet.
5. Time also goes by fast if we have not completed tasks at hand. This causes us to feel stressed. There are a lot of apps that can block certain apps on your phone or on your computer to

minimize your distractions. You can also find apps that track time spent on certain apps and that tell you where you wasted most of your time.

6. I take personal time for rest and relaxation. If I do not feel well rested, I feel miserable and spend extra time doing the same amount of work and feel frustrated. I need my rest to be good at where I am needed as well as what I want to get done.

Journaling Exercise

Here is a journaling exercise for you to immediately put into action some of the strategies you read in this chapter.

    1. What tasks can you delegate?

    2. What tasks can you outsource?

3. What is stopping you from delegating work?

---

4. Where can you add in relaxation to your time?

---

5. Where do you feel you are wasting time the most? What can you do to stop feeling this way?

---

6. Are you using a calendar to help organize your time?

___

7. Do you own a smart device that can remind you of all your important tasks by time?

___

8. Do you use an intention setting exercise daily to finish your main tasks.

___

9. What practices do you know that can help you relax and restore?

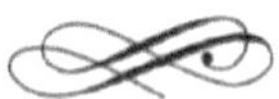

"Follow Your Intuition. It Will Always Take You To The Right Destination." Unknown

Chapter 10

When I say relationship with spirit, you can read it as God, Universe, Higher Self, Grace, or anything else that you like to believe in, or not believe in.. I like all of the mentioned words and I use them all interchangeably. For the purpose of this book, I am going to use the word spirit.

If you know me, one thing you will notice is that I am a constant worrier. My brain is naturally wired (like most people's is) to think the worst possible outcomes of any given situation. And to fixate on the negative outcomes and churn those thoughts constantly in my brain. I am very thankful for the mindful practices I have worked on over the years that prevent me from going insane with these negative thoughts.

One more thing that has helped me prosper is to trust in a power beyond me, that I believe knows more than me, and is always thinking the best for my present and future. This trust in the spirit helps me trust in the overall goodwill in the world, helps me focus on my work, and navigate my stress confidently.

I grew up seeing my mom performing daily rituals. As a child, I thought rituals got in the way of daily busy life, taking time away from the most important things in life. Sometimes, my mom used to make me participate in rituals which I then used to do usually reluctantly.

I had a daily practice of walking to the temple and back home. At the temple, I used to say a prayer and come back home. When I moved to the US, this ritual of walking to the temple stopped completely.

My love for spirituality started blooming. More than rituals, I started learning meditation, reiki, harnessing the power of intuition, mindfulness, Akashic records, sound healing and more. I have learned sudarshan kriya, I have followed Tejguru Sirshree and now I am following the path of kriya yoga. All these learnings have led me to a belief that there is a power beyond me that guides me and shows me the path if I am open to exploring it. It gives me the answers if I am open to hearing them.

I am not asking you to do any of the above.

I am not asking you to follow any particular path or any guru. All I am trying to say is, if you start a daily simple practice of connecting with your inner self, it will help you to trust in your own abilities of navigating your stress. When you trust more, you worry less. When you worry less, you take decisions from a sane mind and that can be an excellent way to get on the path of prosperity.

Practice 1: Gratitude Practice

Since I have started practicing gratitude daily and intentionally, my life perspective on everything has changed. My personal gratitude practice has given me a foundation of optimism that has helped me become a highly self-motivated individual. I have faced a lot of setbacks. My path of growth has been extremely slow and painful. But with the help of gratitude, I have started connecting with opportunities to grow as an entrepreneur.

Simple Gratitude Exercises To Practice Daily

Here are a few exercises that you can practice daily in order to express gratitude and I promise they will take you no time.

Gratitude While Driving In Heavy Traffic– This is an exercise I recommend for those of you who have to deal with heavy traffic and to my husband who has to drive in the wild Atlanta traffic. Just think of three things during the drive that you are feeling thankful for and acknowledge them out loud while in the car.

Create A Gratitude Journal- If you enjoy writing, I recommend carrying a small diary or notebook and noting down at least one sentence daily expressing your gratitude.

Gratitude Meditation– Meditate with gratitude in your heart. Follow this script.

- Find a place to sit down.
- Close your eyes.
- Find a posture that feels relaxed and awake.
- Focus on your breath.

- Drop your shoulders.

- Relax.

- Simply notice what you are experiencing in this moment.

- Maybe you are experiencing a gentle breeze across your face or the comfort of your chair. Maybe you are experiencing some difficulties around what happened earlier today.

- Whatever it is, just notice how you feel inside the body.

- Now slowly shift your awareness towards someone in your life who has supported you in some way.

- It could be your Uber Driver, your mechanic, your teacher, your guru, your parent, your child. Whoever it is, bring them into your awareness.

- Allow yourself to feel how you have benefited from the gift of this being. Allow yourself to feel appreciation and gratitude.

- Now bring awareness to the fact that you are breathing each moment. Knowing that if you are breathing there is more right than wrong. Each breath is a gift of life.

- Allow yourself to notice how precious each breath is. Now slowly open your eyes.

Write A Letter Or A Message– Write a letter expressing heartfelt gratitude to someone in your life that has given you perspective on life, helped you, or has been a blessing.

Create a Gratitude Jar– Write down on pieces of paper what you are grateful for and keep adding them to the jar daily. You can even do this as a family. At the end of the year, you can open the jar and read everything that happened as a blessing throughout the year for you and celebrate the joy

Practice 2: Mindfulness Meditation Practice

The most common misconceptions people have about mindfulness meditation is that they feel the mind should be unwavering and empty from day one. They believe that the mind should get rid of all emotions present. They feel it is all about being a monk and living in caves in the Himalayas. They believe we can immediately achieve a blissful state of mind. The problem with that understanding is that many people get frustrated with the process of meditation. They feel they are doing it wrong because they keep having thoughts and they are trying to attain a "thoughtless" state.

This is where they decide that meditation is not for them. Attaining a thoughtless state, not getting attached to thoughts are all good goals, but not expected to be attained quickly when starting the practice. It takes time and practice.

What is Meditation?

Meditation is the art of being with your thoughts, your breath, yourself, in the present moment.

What is Mindfulness?

Mindfulness is the moment-to-moment experience without judgment. Mindfulness is all about paying attention to the present moment without judging it as good or bad. The true purpose of mindfulness is to rid yourself of needless suffering.

Mindfulness is training for your mind in order to manage it instead of being managed by it.

Beginner's Mindfulness Meditation Practices that I Recommend:

Here are some basic steps to practice five different easy mindfulness meditation practices by yourself. Remember to start in a quiet place free of distractions.

Three Things: Close your eyes and focus on what is around you. Notice three sensations. Notice three sounds. Notice three smells. Then open your eyes. Notice the first three things you see. Notice the first three colors.

Body Scan: Lie or sit comfortably in a relaxed position. Close your eyes. Beginning with your toes and working up throughout your entire body, concentrate on any physical sensations and feelings you are experiencing. Notice any tightness, pain, discomfort, irritation, heat, cold. Once you have reached your head, work your way back down until you reach your toes again. Your job in this exercise is to simply pay attention and be aware of every sensation.

Three Mindful Breaths: Close your eyes. Allow your spine to lift and shoulders to soften. Begin by taking a gentle slow to inhale, resting your attention on the sensation of the air passing over your nostrils and filling your chest and abdomen. Notice the sensations in the body as the air passes back out. Rest for a moment and begin again. Repeat 3 times.

Thought Watching: Close your eyes. Simply notice your thoughts. Avoid judging them. Let the thoughts arise and fall. It is your only duty to notice them. Try not to get carried away with them. If you get carried away with them, you will notice emotions arising. At that moment, bring yourself back to noticing thoughts. You may number the thoughts as they come and go to make it easier for yourself.

5-4-3-2-1: With open eyes, notice five things you can see. Say them loudly or silently in your head. Pause at each one of them and see them completely. Now close your eyes. Notice four things you can feel in the body. Note them to yourself loudly or silently. Now notice and name three things you can hear. Now note two things you can smell. Now finally notice the taste in your mouth. Slowly open your eyes.

Practice 3: Journaling

Something as simple as putting your thoughts to paper has the ability to help you see things more clearly and get an unbiased perspective in life. There are thousands of methods of journaling available on the internet today.

Some types of journaling methods out there are as follows:

1. Dump it all: This method tells you to write down everything that is in your brain on the paper every single day before you begin any task. This helps you start your day with an empty mind.

2. Gratitude journal: Here you list all things you are grateful for. It is designed to help you create more gratitude in your life.

3. Vision Journal: You create a vision board type of a page in every page of this journal with one page dedicated to one goal you want to achieve. This can become an art project and very grounding and fun.

4. One-line journals: Write down a single line every day.

5. Question or Affirmation Journal: You write a question or an affirmation at the top and then continue to elaborate more on that thought in the journal.

There are many more journal types out there. You can follow your own heart and create this reflective and self-nurturing practice which brings you closer to your spirit than ever before.

Practice 4: Pulling Oracle Cards

Now this might sound a little too woo-woo to you, but Oracle cards are one of my favorite ways to connect with intuition and spirit. I do not use Oracle cards to see the future, but I use these cards when I feel stuck in my path and feel that I need extra guidance to move forward.

Oracle cards are a deck of beautifully decorated cards that use different symbols and meanings to share with more insights on your emotions, feelings, your truth and more.

Here are some easy steps to work with an oracle deck:

1. Become very quiet.
2. Ask a question that you want an answer to. An open-ended question like, "What is the message I would like to receive today?" or "What limiting belief may I still be holding on to"?" is better than using something that is a yes or no question or what will happen in your future question.
3. Open the card and look at what message it represents. You can also notice the different symbols and pictures on the card and listen to what images and thoughts they bring up first in your mind. Then go ahead and look at the message that the card producer has associated with the card.

Continuing with this practice helps us find new ways to process our emotions and questions. Oracle cards help with decision making as well as getting a deep insight into your current situation.

Practice 5: Mindful Walking

Whenever I feel frustrated, I take a long, mindful walk. A mindful walk is a walk where you are more aware and in tune with the surroundings and not lost in thoughts. Walking is a great grounding exercise that helps you connect back with your body. Adding mindfulness to the walking helps you connect deeply with your soul while being present in the body. It heightens awareness and enhances your mood.

It is one of the easiest practices or rituals to embody where you do not have to go much out of the way to learn something new. You do not need to buy a journal or oracle deck or learn mindfulness meditations. If you are in doubt, go with this practice. I started with this.

As you enhance your relationship with your inner self, you will find an increased sense of gratitude and less worry developed in yourself. It will build your trust and self-confidence and give you a better outlook towards life. You will naturally vibe high and attract prosperity to you as you wave goodbye to your worries.

Journaling Exercise

Here is a journaling exercise for you to immediately put into action some of the strategies you read in this chapter.

1. Do you currently have a ritual that you use to help enhance your connection with spirit?

2. Which one of the 5 practices called to you the most in this book that you are willing to try?

3. Do you believe in spirit or higher power? Why or Why not?

---

4. What is one thing that you feel most grateful about today?

---

5. Close your eyes and focus on what is around you. Notice three sensations. Notice three sounds. Notice three smells. Then open your eyes. Notice the first three things you see. Notice the first three colors. Write down your experience

---

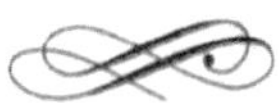

"Knowledge with action converts adversity into prosperity"
APJ Abdul Kalam

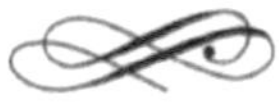

SECTION 2

THE PATH TO PROSPERITY

Chapter 11

Integration of Knowledge of The Houses and Moving Towards Prosperity

In the first section, we have learned a lot about prosperity and what triggers us to move away from prosperity and towards stress. I hope that you have journaled quite a bit on all these houses of prosperity to really understand how every area of life is extremely important to maintain a balance and understand how prosperity is not just about money.

I want you to take a deep breath here and really go back and journal at the end of each chapter if you have not done so already. I want you to make sure that you understand the houses of prosperity clearly.

I know that if you are reading this book, you probably have read a lot of self-help books or management books. Knowing and reading is important. But what really makes a difference is taking action.

Implementation is key. I want this book to be life changing for you. I want to see you prosper. And this might seem harsh, more like a school principal, making sure that kids are doing their homework. I have no problem being a little harsh right now because I know this little push can help you.

Once you are done taking action on earlier chapters, I invite you to implement what you read in the next section. The next section focuses on the "Path to Prosperity." My goal in writing it was to teach you the exact steps that you can take to find prosperity in each of the ten houses. You can just follow this same process in each house and you will always be able to find your way to abundance and joy for that house.

I was very excited to share the process in this book and I am sure you will love it and would want to implement it right away. Carry on reading.

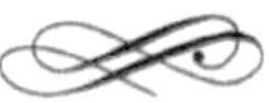

"There is no way to prosperity, prosperity is the way."
Wayne Dyer

Chapter 12

Four Steps To Prosperity

All books on prosperity and abundance point to one thing.- Maintain the feeling of abundance in the present moment to attract more prosperity. Wayne Dyer says so. Rhonda Bryne says so. Eckhart Tolle says so. My gurus say so.

While this seems so simple, it is not an easy task for everyone. If it was, more people would feel prosperous and there would not be a need to write this book.

But instead, stress prevails and that is why I feel the need to write down a step-by-step path to prosperity which goes beyond just the feelings. It gives you a practical approach to live your life with abundance and prosperity day after day after day.

But before I share the path with you, let me tell you my story of our house in Atlanta.

In 2004, I read a book called Synchro-Destiny by Deepak Chopra, that talked about life's synchronicities. I found it very interesting, learning about humans having an energy and how these energies affect each other. I learned how a simple butterfly fluttering its wings in one area can create thunderstorms in another. I loved the idea of how synchronicities play a part in everything in our life. I did not make much of it until much later in my life.

In 2016, we were living in Las Vegas. What we thought was going to be a 4 year thing, had become a 6 year thing and we saw no signs of moving anywhere outside of Las Vegas. While we loved living there, we were looking forward to a change of scenery, to move out and explore opportunities in different states.

We were frustrated and unhappy in a lot of ways because of this. In late 2016, I came across the founder of Infinite Receiving, Maru Iabichella. How I ended up in her live program as an attendee was a synchronicity in itself. In one of her videos, she taught a process on visualizing the future.

So I started visualizing myself, drinking a cup of Indian tea (masala chai) on a deck that looks over a lawn and there are some trees at the horizon. Since

Vegas was so brown, I was looking forward to moving to a greener space. So, with the intention of the possibility of a move, I created this visualization and enjoyed it. While we were feeling anxious, desperate, and sometimes frustrated about our situation, this intention gave me great joy.

In a few weeks of this visualization, my husband got a few interview calls out of Nevada. While on an interview, he got another interview call from Atlanta. And somehow this Atlanta thing worked out and we were there in four weeks. Guess where there are decks with greenery and trees and basement? In Atlanta!

In 2 months of moving to Atlanta, I was on that deck similar to the one that I visualized with a cup of tea in my hand!

If I look back at how I met my husband, how we moved to Vegas, how I ended up doing sound healing and meditation retreats, and how I ended up writing this book it all follows the exact same sequence of steps.

These 4 Steps make the path for stress-free prosperity. If you consciously open up to it, it will change your life, just like it has changed mine.

Four Steps To Stress - Free Prosperity

1. Set an intention

Setting an intention means writing down a short positive statement or a blessing for yourself. Setting an intention can be a form of prayer or guideline that you create for yourself that shows you how your life, your relationship with yourself, your relationships with different houses of prosperity should look like.

Is there a difference between setting an intention and setting a goal?

Yes, there is a slight difference. When you are setting goals, they can come from someone else or from you and they usually include detailed plans of actions ideally resulting in how you will go about achieving those goals. They are more about achieving something. Goals are more specific, exact even. Intentions are more generalized.

For example, your career goal can be becoming a partner in your law firm by age 42. Your intention for your career can be something on the lines of

"Through my work, I protect humanity and its values,." or "I always prosper as my clients prosper."

Your intentions come from your heart. They reflect your values. They become your guiding principles and help you hold on to your values.

2. Pay Attention To Synchronicities

As I said before, it took me years to really understand what I read in Deepak Chopra's book. I believe it is a synchronicity that led me down the path of reading the book and one day, writing about it in my own book that highlights synchronicities. When you pay attention to synchronicities happening in the moment, your excitement about your life will light up and you will be led to a path of opportunities that will fulfill your intention.

It is your duty to understand and recognize these moments. Has it ever happened to you that you wrote down something and the next thing you know, someone calls you and tells you a similar story that highlights what you wrote down? Happens a lot, right? That is synchronicity.

Synchronicity is a coincidence, a series of unexplained seemingly related events (that have no explainable direct relation) that happen after one event.

In our case, our first event is writing down our intention. Synchronicities follow intention. They always do. All you have to do is notice them on purpose and with intention.

Here are some examples of synchronicity in action.

- Your intention is to be more useful today. And your neighbor knocks on your door and asks you for help.
- Or your intention is to make money and you get mail with a credit limit increase.
- Or you set an intention to notice beauty and you find the most beautiful bird perched right on your front porch.

The more you write down these intentions and notice your synchronicities, the more you will find yourself on the path to prosperity.

3. Take an Inspired Action

When we write down goals, we usually have a series of action steps or to-do lists written down. But when you set an intention, your inspired action will be an action that will jump to you as the next thing to do following the synchronicity.

For example, once I wrote down as an intention, "I am thankful for all the friendships in my life." Interestingly, the moment I kept my pen down, someone messaged me and said they wanted to connect with me and invite me for tea. Now here is where the inspired action comes in. I was inspired to say yes to this new friend because I had just written about friendships.

An inspired action is just that. An action that comes to you in the moment of time as an inspiration. That does not mean you leave your to-do lists aside.

It means that you give importance to the synchronicity and take that inspired action and do it right away.

4. Let go

What does letting go mean? Letting go does not mean not taking action. Letting go does not mean not expecting the result.

Letting go means not having an emotional attachment to the outcome or the process of how prosperity enters your life.

This step is the trickiest step of all. It is never clear to most people how to let go. In this book, I have simplified the letting go process and exactly set it for you to be able to follow it step by step. Let's keep reading!

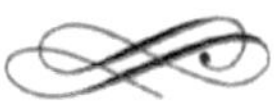

"If danger arises in the present moment, there may be an emotion.

There may even be pain. But that's a challenge, not a problem. For a problem to exist, you need time and repetitive mind activity." Eckhart Tolle

Chapter 13

S tress Free Prosperity is a simple roadmap to a prosperous life. It is a systematic step by step formula to help people create a stress-free prosperous life.

Still, a lot of people will get stuck. And they will all get stuck in this one area: Letting Go of outcomes.

We get attached to what we want in our life so much that we start walking the path of self-sabotage. When we are too attached to our goals and intentions, we become desperate to see results. We stop trusting our alignment, our abilities and we refuse to let nature play its role.

This puts us in the mindset of F.R.A.W.D.S.

Meet The F.R.A.W.D.S

When we decide to step up and do something that is out of our normal comfort zone, we see that we are thrown a curveball sometimes and we have to overcome a great deal of mental resistance before we move forward. This mental block is a result of extreme conditioning of our belief systems, past experiences, and expectations.

We will dive into the reasons later but let us introduce you to the F.R.A.W.D.S first.

Meet F:

F stands for **FEAR**. In the path of our life, we face fears daily. Fear of dying, fear of heights, fear of losing our loved ones, fear of not making it to the top, fear of animals and insects, fear of this and fear of that.

Fear shows up to help you not change at all. It wants everything to stay the same and have you live the same protected life all the time. It leads to creating anxiety in your system if left uncontrolled. And a lot of times, our lizard brain creates that fear (Lizard brain is the part of the brain to which primitive, nonrational, or self-interested behavior is attributed. It is responsible for primitive survival instincts such as aggression and fear).

Fear of rejection is a quite common fear for those in the public eye, when we approach the person of our dreams, or apply to the dream job. Deep-rooted under the fear is a conditioning of low self-esteem that may have occurred due to past trauma, abuse, accident, etc.

I had a fear of public speaking. I could deliver presentations to a handful of colleagues at work with ease. However, since I left work and decided to step into the world of spiritual and personal development, I realized that my fear would make it hard for me to get up and just start talking on this subject. I wondered if people would ridicule me for not having authority on the subject. I wondered if I would be ridiculed for being a novice.

The fun part is synchronicity had something else in store for me. I received a free ticket to go to a conference. In that conference, people were asked what their biggest dream was and what was stopping them from doing that. I raised my hand and said, I want to share my voice like famous people do on stage but I am incredibly scared of public speaking.

At that moment, I was called on stage to say that very sentence again. It was hard for me to admit this fear in front of hundreds of people. I also realized that in that moment, while saying that sentence, I had faced my fear of public speaking while sharing my deepest truth. And I was still alive. I cried on stage. But after that, sharing my voice daily became much easier.

I went on to create an online interview summit and interviewed 35 entrepreneurial women on how they handle self-care and business. A lot of those women were also single moms running successful businesses and taking care of their children and themselves. It was an eye opener and gave me more courage to navigate my fears.

One of those people that I interviewed was my first entrepreneurial friend Sara. Sara is a brave woman. She has volunteered in war zones and helped people with trauma and abuse while things were bad. She is a single mother and shows courage every day in her life. When I mentioned my fears to her, she told me something that has stuck with me ever since.

She told me that courage is not the absence of fear. Courage means moving forward despite fear. Everyone has fear. They do great things anyway. I think in my scary entrepreneurial world, these lines have become my holy grail. I have stepped up and faced fears daily and so do most people who decide to change their life for the better, who decide to stand up and share their truth, those who decide to challenge the authorities, those who stand in the middle of nowhere and fight for the country. All of them are facing fears.

F from the F.R.A.W.D.S. will never go away. It is up to you to recognize this and move on despite it. It is up to you to tame it and make it your friend. It is up to you to call it out and then move on keeping it on your side.

The caveat here though is that we also need to acknowledge that at times fear helps you and rightfully so. Fear is our brain trying to keep us safe.

The problem shows up when we get worked up about our fear and get paralyzed. That is when our *not really a friend* R shows.

Meet R:

RESISTANCE is your mind's inertia to help you be safe. Rooted inside resistance is fear of change. We are afraid that things might not be the same after taking action.

Our mind is programmed to keep us safe from the wildlife outside our caves. This means resisting even the smallest of action that leads us away from the safety of the cave. And even if we have transformed so much from a wild cave man to a sophisticated species through the industrial and technological age, our primal instincts keep us safe from the unknown, the unseen and the unexperienced.

We, as a society, must learn ways to understand this programming and then actively work on changing these functions.

Overcoming resistance is not a day at the beach. But sometimes when you have all the work to do, you instead decide to pack your bags and go to the beach.

Look inside your heart and see if there is any resistance. If you are working on A which is your priority, but your mind starts nagging you about how B and C are more important and you end up pushing all work out and not doing anything, you will know with your soul that you are facing strong internal resistance.

Meet A:

A is for **ANGER.** Anger is a surface emotion of annoyance, displeasure or hostility that takes too much space and energy away from us. We are filled with rage about worldly news, about our needs not being met, about how something happened to us and so on.

Take your attention to this phrase again - "surface emotion". Inside of anger, hidden could be grief, unmet needs of love and attention, feelings of helplessness or loss of control, and feelings of being wronged.

When we focus on anger, it only grows. We give fuel to our angry thoughts by regurgitating them and acting upon them. The problem is anger only gives rise to hurt feelings, more anger and moves us further away from any feelings of prosperity.

WORRY and Anxiety pretty much go hand in hand. Worry is more specific about a certain situation and temporary while anxiety is vague. Worry tends to affect our thoughts while anxiety tends to affect our body and mind.

If you decide that you will let Fear and Resistance run your life, then you will be the one that is facing **ANXIETY and WORRY.**

The basis of this feeling is that you are not feeling safe.

When you have too much fear and resistance, you keep churning those thoughts. This is because in one way you want to give life a better response and change, but on the other hand your resistance will not let you. It will keep showing you scary pictures of how life is going to be bad and not great and how you might lose everything. And when our mind falls for that repeatedly, our anxiety trips us.

Fear and resistance will always be there in our life. If you are trying to make anxiety go away and disappear, it is not going to work. Fear and resistance cannot disappear completely.

It is for us to recognize that life is not controlled by us. What we can control is only the response we give to life. By bringing our reactions under control, we can control fear and resistance.

We live in a constant world of uncertainty. When we are faced with uncertainty, we do not know how to react to what is going to happen. We worry about the future. We worry about what people will think of us. We worry what will happen to our children.

The one thing we must realize when it comes to worry is that, when we worry, it is a given that the outcome is not in our control. So, our constant worrying is not going to matter much.

A lot of books and self-help people try to teach us on how to remove the bad things from our lives. Instead, I am trying to show you that you do not focus your energy on things that you cannot control. Things that invoke fear and resistance are mere signals in life that help you respond better to life.

Meet D:

D stands for **DESPERATION.** When we really want something, we get attached to the outcome. We get so attached that we cannot think of anything else. We keep obsessing about it. This is where there is a thin line between attracting something and repelling something out of our zone.

When desperation happens, you start taking action from a place of lack and disbelief. Many times, desperation leads to ineffective actions and pushes us in the wrong direction. It creates self - sabotage.

Meet S:

SHAME is an emotion that plagues us all. Shame of not having enough. Shame of being late to achieve something. Shame of losing. Shame of doing something that we were not supposed to do. Shame comes from an extreme judgement of ourselves and sometimes from society. It is deep rooted in our society. Shame researcher, Brene Brown says, *"Shame is the most powerful, master emotion. It's the fear that we're not good enough."*

On the road to prosperity, just meeting with the F.R.A.W.D.S is not enough. They can take us in a deep depressive state. We must work on dealing with them.

When we are dealing with life's stress, we want to know that we are still in control.

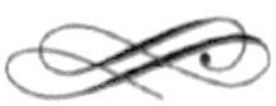

*"I still sometimes feel like a loser kid in high school
and I just have to pick myself up and tell myself that
I'm a superstar every morning so that I can get
through this day and be for my fans what they need for
me to be."*

Lady Gaga

Chapter 14

S tress tends to take our control away. When we are stressed out, we find ourselves reacting to everything. We get into a cycle of chaos, confusion, and worry. All we really want to know in that time of deep stress, and point of no return, is that there is a light that we can see to come back to our normal selves.

I am listing some simple steps to help you get started with recognizing and dealing with your fears, your resistance, your anger, your worries, your desperation, and your shame.

I learned these steps through a series of failures, stress, and hard times, wins and good times but most importantly through my support system that I found through my husband, my sister, my mother and father, my gurus, my coaches and teachers, through mindfulness, through prayer and meditation, through energy healing and coaching sessions with my clients and some through my children.

1. Acknowledge your stress and name the F.R.A.W.D.S

I have a long experience in the manufacturing and process industry as an Industrial Engineer. I have been on hundreds of problem-solving projects. The first thing we ever do in order to solve a problem is to define it correctly.

When you define the exact problem, you are able to look in the right direction and ask the right questions. For example, if a production conveyor line went down, we first asked what exactly caused the machine line to be down. The production conveyor line was down as an outcome but what was the first thing that seemingly caused it is the main problem. If we found out that the XYZ machine on the conveyor broke down, we had a definite problem to go after instead of looking at the whole conveyor belt.

Similarly in real life, when we are stressed out, just saying that we are stressed out, is not going to help.

Finding out which one of the **F.R.A.W.D.S** is causing the issue and naming it is very important.

You can start by filling in the blanks of any or all of these sentences to find out what is really bothering you.

1. I feel ………………
2. I am angry because……………
3. I am worried that……………..
4. I am ashamed of…………..
5. I really need……………….
6. I am afraid that……………

2. Process Your Emotions

Before we shift into feeling positive, it is necessary to process emotions. The one thing that emotions really want is for their presence to be acknowledged, accepted, and heard.

Emotions are less about reactions and more about understanding. Growing up, we have always seen adults reacting in different ways that are not exactly the healthiest ways to deal with our emotions.

Processing emotions is a learned skill and unfortunately not many people teach it openly.

Here are some ways that you can process your emotions:

1. **Noticing your emotions within**: An easy way to process any emotion is to go within and notice it in the body. In mindfulness practices, we close our eyes and invite emotions to arise. We try to pinpoint where in the body we are feeling this emotion. And then we breathe through this emotion and let it arise. We listen to see what this emotion has to say to us. We listen to our hidden beliefs and stories. And breathe through this. We thank the emotion for showing up and sharing the truth.
2. **Crying it out**: Sometimes just crying it out can help the excess stress hormones like cortisol release, which in turn provides a calming effect.
3. **Journaling**: Dumping all that is in your mind onto a piece of paper can help your brain to transfer the stress on to the paper.

Once your brain knows that you have your stress written down, it will not keep reminding you about it all the time. It assumes you will be doing something about it. Daily journaling practice is an excellent way to process emotions.

4. **Voice your emotions**- When we voice our emotions, we are able to express and hear what is really bothering us. Doing this in a safe space like that in the presence of a coach, a therapist or a trusted friend can provide us deep compassion that we need when we are feeling low.

3. What is in your control and what is not in your control?

A lot of times, everything that we worry about is not in our control. But some things are. When you find out what you are stressed about, the next step is to understand your current role in your situation.

Once we process our emotions, it is easy to distinguish what is in our control and what is not in our control anymore.

Asking these questions can help:

1. Is there anything I can actively do about this situation? Is it in my control?
2. What about this situation is not in my control? Will any action that I take affect my situation at all?

One of my close friends pointed something to me once when I apologized for getting late. She said that once you are already late, there is not much that you can do actively any more to get there on time. So might as well drive safe and not hurry.

There was so much wisdom in those words. It can be applied to any situation. We have to focus only on and immediately address what is in our power and let go of what is not.

In this situation, what was in my control was calling my friend and telling her I will be late and driving safe. I had lost control already on getting there in time. So, worrying about getting late was not going to get me anywhere other than feeling guilty and shameful.

Stress happens the most when things start to get out of your control zone.

This is where our lizard brain kicks in and keeps telling us that there is danger, and we must work on it. We get into fight or flight mode. This is where most of us give in to the stress and start feeling the anxiety, the anger, frustration, the fear of what is next, the urge to quit it all and a lot more.

4. Elicit the relaxation response

"Relaxation response" is a term coined by Dr. Herbert Benson, in his book The Relaxation Response. The relaxation response is defined as the personal ability to elicit the rest and digest phase or the parasympathetic nervous system.

This response naturally reduces physical stress, improves sleep, increases resilience, relieves pains, enhances mood and does so much more.

This is not just done by shutting off and going to sleep, but by following techniques that will actively calm your brain and ease your stress.

There are a number of ways you can elicit the relaxation response. My favorite ways are through pranayama, yoga nidra, sound healing, mindfulness, and restorative yoga. I share these with my clients through private practice as well as on my social media and YouTube channels. Once you have given enough space for your emotions to be released, your stress to be released, your relaxation to set in, and you will create a way for feeling prosperous and joyful. When you take actions and set intentions from this space of expansiveness, you will naturally see results, you will flourish and more importantly you will enjoy the journey.

If you keep just wishing for things to change, keep faking your joy and your feelings, you will not go anywhere except round and round in circles.

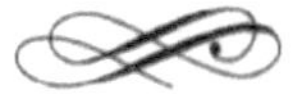

"I like cancelled plans. And empty bookstores. I like rainy days and thunderstorms. And quiet coffee shops. I like messy beds and over-worn pajamas. Most of all, I like the small joys that a simple life brings."

Unknown

Chapter 15

Conclusion

Most of us will be upset if thunderstorms cancel our plans, if our beds are messy daily and the bookstores do not carry our favorite books.

The idea of stress-free prosperity is to process these feelings of stress in the moment and then come back to the very thing that relaxes you and puts you in a better mood to handle your day.

How is this done is through daily practice?

The daily practice of setting intentions, the daily practice of noticing synchronicities, the daily practice of dealing with your negative emotions, the daily practice of taking inspired actions is what you need to deal with the stress.

When you intentionally start working on your daily prosperity practice, you will be more in control of your stress and relaxation hormones and will be less reactive to situations around you.

It does not matter which house of prosperity is upside down, your daily routine is the key to bring it back. This helps you win daily. And when you win daily, you find yourself on the road to stress free prosperity.

What are you waiting for?

I have laid down the exact plan for you to deal with your stress and get to the other side. It is now your turn to start implementing what you learned in this book. That is the key. That is where you will see results.

If you read this book and throw it in the trash, return it to the store, re-sell it, gift it to your friend, give it back to the library or decorate your shelf with it, it will not help you. What will help you is holding yourself accountable daily to practice what you read.

It is in your hands to not become part of a statistic for stress. As I said before, a lot of people complain about their stress. Only a few people do something about it. It is completely up to you.

Will you become a statistic, or will you do something about it? The ball is now in your court.